·四川大学精品立项教材·

ADVANCES IN LABORATORY MEDICINE

检验医学进展

主　审　应斌武　秦　莉　江　虹

主　编　康　梅

副主编　陈　捷　谢　轶　何　超

编　委　（按姓氏拼音排序）

白杨娟　蔡　蓓　蔡俊君　干　伟

何　詠　廖红艳　武永康　王立新

叶远馨　郑　沁

四川大学出版社
SICHUAN UNIVERSITY PRESS

项目策划：龚娇梅
责任编辑：龚娇梅
责任校对：张　澄
封面设计：墨创文化
责任印制：王　炜

图书在版编目（CIP）数据

检验医学进展 = Advances in Laboratory Medicine：
英文 / 康梅主编．— 成都：四川大学出版社，2021.7
四川大学精品立项教材
ISBN 978-7-5690-4832-2

Ⅰ．①检… Ⅱ．①康… Ⅲ．①医学检验－高等学校－
教材－英文 Ⅳ．① R446

中国版本图书馆 CIP 数据核字（2021）第 144462 号

书名	ADVANCES IN LABORATORY MEDICINE
主　　编	康　梅
出　　版	四川大学出版社
地　　址	成都市一环路南一段 24 号（610065）
发　　行	四川大学出版社
书　　号	ISBN 978-7-5690-4832-2
印前制作	四川胜翔数码印务设计有限公司
印　　刷	成都金龙印务有限责任公司
成品尺寸	185mm×260mm
插　　页	4
印　　张	10.5
字　　数	348 千字
版　　次	2021 年 12 月第 1 版
印　　次	2021 年 12 月第 1 次印刷
定　　价	49.00 元

◆ 读者邮购本书，请与本社发行科联系。
　电话：(028)85408408/(028)85401670/
　(028)86408023　邮政编码：610065
◆ 本社图书如有印装质量问题，请寄回出版社调换。
◆ 网址：http://press.scu.edu.cn

四川大学出版社
微信公众号

ACKNOWLEDGEMENTS

Thank all the persons who participated in the writing, revising and publishing of this book. Thank all the teachers who participated in the professional English teaching of the Department of Laboratory Medicine, West China school of Medicine, Sichuan University.

CONTENTS

CHAPTER 1

INTRODUCTION TO LABORATORY MEDICINE

1 *Words and phrases*

Laboratory medicine　检验医学

Auxiliary　辅助的

Metabolism　代谢

Faculty　员工

Immunology　免疫学

Biochemistry　生物化学

Genetics　遗传学

Hematology　血液学

Ecsomatics　体液检验学

Molecular diagnosis　分子诊断学

Microbiology　微生物学

Virology　病毒学

Residents　住院医生

Accuracy　准确度

Prognosis　预后

Discipline　学科

Practitioner　从业者

Epoch-making　划时代的

Physiology　生理学

Etiology　病因学，病原学

Rickettsia　立克次体

Qualitative　定性的

Quantitative　定量的

Ultrastructure　超微结构

Parasitology　寄生虫学

Preclinical medicine　基础医学

Electrophoresis　电泳

Hemoglobin electrophoresis　血红蛋白电泳

Flame photometer　火焰光度计

Indirect hemagglutination test　间接血凝试验

Latex agglutination experiment　乳胶凝集试验

Gas chromatograph　气相色谱仪

Double diffusion test　双向扩散试验

Unilateral diffusion test　单向扩散试验

Counterpimmunoelectrophoresis　对流免疫电泳

Fluorescence polarization　荧光偏振

Fluorescence immunoassay　荧光免疫测定

Chemiluminescence　化学发光

Biosensor　生物传感器

Biochip　生物芯片

Amniotic fluid　羊水

Exfoliated cells　脱落细胞

Mycology　真菌学

Immunolabeling technology　标记免疫技术

Enzyme-linked immunosorbent assay　酶联免疫吸附试验

Ratenephelometry　速率散射比浊

Eugenics　优生优育

Polymerase chain reaction　聚合酶链反应

Liquid mass spectrometry　液相质谱仪

2　Readings

Laboratory medicine is an auxiliary diagnostic discipline, which originated from the integration of modern laboratory technology and clinical medicine, also known as experimental diagnostics. Through the use of modern physical and chemical methods and means, it is an important discipline for medical diagnosis of patients.

The department of laboratory medicine can provide leading edge clinical care, outstanding biomedical research and comprehensive education. Technologists established methodologies for the rigorous examination of the chemical composition of blood and urine that brought quantitative discipline to the study of human metabolism. This department typically has faculties involved in basic and clinical work. Their routine research work focusing on immunology, biochemistry, advanced therapy, biomarker discovery, cancer and molecular genetics, data science (computational healthcare and imaging), microbiology, virology, etc. Faculties are also involved in teaching residents, medical students, graduate students.

Laboratory investigations are performed and the results of laboratory tests are made available to patients through their clinicians. Clinical advice is available on the ordering of examinations and the interpretation of examination results. Advanced laboratory technologies are used to provide results more quickly, accurately and comprehensively. Laboratory medicine is useful and important for clinical diagnosis, treatment and prognosis assessment.

2.1   History, current situation and progress of laboratory medicine

With the tide of scientific and technological progress, the rapid development of medicine, and related disciplines, some small and scattered clinical laboratories managed by doctors have developed into more centralized laboratories with specialized practitioners and equipments, and gradually formed the clinical laboratory discipline. Over the past two decades, advanced development of clinical medicine greatly promoted the clinicians to pay attention to its related area (e. g. pathology, laboratory medicine). Biological samples such as hormones play an important physiological role in clinical diagnosis, but the concentration of such materials is very low. Therefore, we are facing the challenge to provide rapid and sensitive test.

Since the 18th century when Leeuwenhoek used a homemade microscope to see bacteria, microbial etiology was established and the emerging discipline of bacteriology began to sprout. Due to the joint efforts of bacteriologists, scientists have a new understanding of pathogenic bacteria, rickettsia, virus, and have establish new concepts, such as microbiology and immunology. Since the 1820s, biochemistry has gradually developed into an independent discipline, conducting in-depth research on the material metabolism and energy conversion of human proteins, lipids, sugars, and vitamins, and establishing the basic theory of biochemistry as well as qualitative and quantitative detection methods of various chemical substances in human body. At the beginning of the 20th century, biologists carried out a lot of research work on protein in the blood, immune and nutrition, because the ultrastructure widely used in the field of medicine, blood cytology and pathology, human parasitology, gradually developed into preclinical medicine, thus laid a foundation for the formation of the comprehensive science. By the mid-1980s, laboratory medicine has made great improvement in our country, in terms of hematology, in addition to the blood cell count and morphological examination, coagulation test and hemolysis test were widely used, electronic automatic blood count method , hemoglobin electrophoresis and subcellular structure have been used in clinical laboratories.

In biological chemistry, in addition to various biochemical material qualitative and quantitative detection in blood or other body fluids, liver and kidney function tests are established, and the protein electrophoresis, enzymes, hormones and other complex detections are used for clinical diagnosis, many labs have used flame photometer, ultraviolet spectrophotometer, blood gas analyzer, optical density meter and automatic biochemical analyzer, etc. gradually, single reagent was used to quick analysis, application of isotope labeling biological immune and other new technologies were developed.

In microbiology, technologists carried out pathogenic bacteria cultivation and bacteria identification, antimicrobial susceptibility test and combined susceptibility test. They used medium immuno-fluorescence technology for rapid diagnosis, small bottles of cultivation technology, anaerobic membrane, cultivate membrane filtration technology. They have developed isolation, identification, and culture of the various virus. Automatic analysis instruments were used to perform rapid identification of bacteria and antimicrobial susceptibility test.

In immune serology, technologists have carried out various antigen-antibody indirect hemagglutination tests, latex agglutination experiment, plasma cell immunity, humoral immunity testing, immune diffusion, electrophoresis and fluorescence immune and enzyme label, all kinds of precipitation reaction and complement fixation, and the determination of immune complex. electron microscope, spectrophotometer, optical density scanner, gas chromatograph, atomic absorption spectrometer, blood acid-base balance, liquid scintillation counter, electronic automatic blood cell counter, biochemical automatic analyzer, etc. , were widely used by the mid − 1980s, then foreign laboratory medicine developed to a higher level of automation and microscale.

In terms of clinical examination equipment, the development of electronic technology, especially the application of microcomputer in laboratory medicine, makes clinical examination to develop towards the direction of automation, multiple, rapid, micro and accurate, This realizes mechanization, automation, multiple trace fast biochemical test. They made the development of high precision, automation instrument from single-channel to multi-channel, the kinds of up to 12 to 24 pipe joint analysis of device, detect the 24 biochemical test results. At the same time, they combined several fixed examination, which could determinate thousands of specimens in each hour.

With the continuous efforts of many scholars, great progress was made in the field of microbiology, such as bacterial smear with antibodies, and acid dye fast assay methods, enrichment culture and raising the temperature, to shorten the time, improve the positive rate, as well as speed up the determination of pathogenic bacteria sensitivity to drugs. In serology and immunology, scientists discovered some new antigenic determinants, depending on the function of cell membrane receptors and classifying cells, and tested percentage distribution and function of each group of cells. They established double diffusion test, unilateral diffusion test, counter immunoelectrophoresis, rocket electrophoresis, indirect agglutination test, reverse indirect agglutination, and complement fixation test, etc. Tumor immunity and pathological tissue antigen-antibody diagnostic and the immunoglobulin determination provided new ways to assess disease progress.

The application of advanced and new technologies, such as fluorescence polarization, chemiluminescence, molecular markers, biosensor, and biochip, has not only led to the development of clinical testing instruments and equipment with higher sensitivity, less sample volume, faster analysis speed and more convenient operation, but also shortened the renewal period of testing instruments. The realization of "modularization" and "completed laboratory automation" of clinical test instruments breaks the traditional technical division of labor mode of clinical test, and makes a sample automatically complete all the requirements of different test items such as hematology, biochemistry, and immunity. The miniaturization and simplicity of clinical testing instruments enable laboratory staffs, clinicians, nurses, and even patients' own relatives to perform tests at patients' bedsides or patients' homes, not need specialized laboratories anymore.

In the clinical application, laboratory analysis of human samples by microbiology, immunology, biochemistry, genetics, hematology, biophysics, cytology, and other aspects of the test, could provide patients with suggestions for prevention, diagnosis, treatment evaluation. Nowadays, more and more new medical technologies are also applied to laboratory medicine. In the 1990s, great changes and leaps have taken place in clinical testing, from "medical testing" to "laboratory medicine". This change has also made technologists more clearly aware of their tasks and challenges. In addition, new medical equipment, medical technology and new natural science also have more stringent requirements on laboratory medicine.

Laboratory medicine has entered a new chapter with the development of the whole medical cause. The transformation or characteristics of laboratory medicine in China can be summed up in eight aspects: automation, miniaturization (family), molecularization, internationalization, standardization, personalization, networking, and informatization. Entering the 21st century, the development of natural science has promoted the development of medicine. Medical examination greatly changes from the original manual operation to more computer-controlled automation. In terms of content, the emergence of new technologies and methods, such as molecular biology technology and immune labeling technology, has given new content and new development space for medical testing.

2. 2   Branches and functions of laboratory medicine

Clinical laboratory medicine using the conventional testing methods of invitro blood, urine, feces, reproductive system secretions, cerebrospinal fluid, serous cavity effusion, specimens of amniotic fluid, and exfoliated cells, such as chemistry, biology, morphology, provide an important basis for disease diagnosis, monitoring, and treatment. In the clinical department of laboratory medicine, clinical hematology is usually included in the same division of basic laboratory examination. It mainly studies the pathological and physiological processes of the occurrence and evolution of hematopoietic tissues and blood cells, uses various laboratory examination methods and techniques to analyze the pathological changes of blood and hematopoietic organs, to clarify the occurrence mechanism of blood diseases, assist in diagnosis, treatment observation, and prognosis judgment.

The scope of work in clinical hematology includes routine blood cell analysis, reticulocyte count, erythrocyte sedimentation rate and classification count of white blood cells, etc. Relevant tests for anticoagulation, related tests for hemolysis, functional tests for platelets, and thromboelastogram are also determined in this division. It provides strong laboratory evidence for the diagnosis of diseases related to bleeding and clotting. Routine urine dry chemical and sediment analysis, stool routine and occulted blood, semen examination, all kinds of body fluid routine and other special items examination are also included. Technologists in this area are familiar with blood morphology in bone marrow cells, chemical staining and leukemia cell immune classification analysis. Good at integrating the use of the WHO classification criteria and principles of MICM classification of various blood system diseases diagnosis, they could provide medical staff with powerful laboratory evidence for treatment, monitoring, and prognosis assessment. In recent years, the division of hematology focuses their research work on the prevention, control, and management of thrombotic diseases, the mechanism research and clinical diagnosis of malignant tumors in the blood system, platelets and their role in inflammatory diseases, etc. In the field of hematology, more and more new technologies gradually emerge, such as automatic reading, artificial intelligence interpretation of morphological results, automatic report check, etc., expanding the space for the development of this specialty.

Clinical biochemistry test uses chemical and biochemical techniques to detect human specimens, analyze the composition and metabolism of substances under specific physiological and pathological conditions, and provides a basis for the prevention, diagnosis, treatment, and prognosis of clinical diseases. A cross-discipline developed gradually by the cross-integration of chemistry, biochemistry, clinical medicine, and other disciplines. It includes diagnostic enzymology in the biochemical examination, biochemical examination of substance metabolism and internal environmental disorders, major organ system diseases and special physiological phenomena, biochemical examination of pregnancy, monitoring of therapeutic drug concentration, application, and evaluation of biochemical automatic analyzer, quality control, etc.

Clinical biochemistry analyzes liver function, renal function, blood glucose, electrolytes, blood lipid, enzymology, body fluids and urine biochemical, blood gas analysis, serum protein electrophoresis, pituitary hormones and cardiac markers, thyroid hormones and related antibodies, parathyroid and bone metabolism-related hormones, gonadal hormones, adrenal hormones, diabetes-related projects. Besides the above routine biochemical items, serum iron, total iron-binding capacity, plasma lactic acid, blood ammonia, plasma ethanol and other items are also provided. In recent years, the divisions of biochemistry focus their research work on mechanisms and new biomarkers of endocrine and metabolic diseases, liver and kidney diseases, and cardiovascular diseases.

Clinical microbiology is a branch that identifies the pathogens from clinical samples to guide management and treatment strategies for patients with infections. It has been divided into several divisions, including bacteriology, virology, mycology, etc. Nowadays, diagnostic techniques in clinical microbiology include microscopic examination, isolation and culture of microorganisms, antimicrobial susceptibility test, detection of pathogen specific antibodies (serology) or antigens, molecular identification of microbial nucleic acids (DNA or RNA), and the newly-developed techniques (e. g. metagenomic approaches). Also, clinical microbiology can provide the consultant of the reports, surveil the antimicrobial susceptibility of the isolates in each local setting, and assume the paramount role in the antimicrobial stewardship.

Clinical immunology test is using immune detection principle and technology, to analyze immune active cells, antigen and antibody, complement, cytokines, cell adhesion molecules, immune-related trace substances in the body fluids, such as hormones, enzymes, plasma, trace protein, blood drug concentration, trace elements, for clinical diagnosis analysis of condition adjustment, treatment, and prognosis, etc. Immunology technology with the development of immunolabeling technology has made a great leap. With the rapid development of monoclonal antibody technology and computer application technology, fluorescence immunoassay, enzyme-linked immunoassay, rate nephelometry, chemiluminescence immunoassay, flow cytometry and western blotting assay have been applied to clinical laboratories. Good specificity, high sensitivity, simplicity, rapidity and stability make them irreplaceable in clinical diagnosis, treatment, prevention, and research.

Clinical immunology also detects humoral immunity, cellular immunity, infection immunity, cytokines, tumor markers, autoantibodies, allergen screening, therapeutic drug monitoring, poison screening, etc. In recent years, the division of immunology focuses research work on mechanisms of autoimmune diseases, such as systemic lupus erythematosus, rheumatoid arthritis, cellular immune regulation in the tumor, transplantation, infectious diseases, etc.

Molecular diagnostics is based on the theory of molecular biology, using the techniques and methods of molecular biology to study the existence, structure, or expression regulation of endogenous or exogenous biological macromolecules in the human body, to provide information and decision basis for disease prevention, prediction, diagnosis, treatment, and prognosis. It uses molecular biological methods to detect changes in the structure or expression level of genetic material in patients. Molecular diagnosis is the main method of prediction diagnosis, which can be used for individual genetic disease diagnosis and prenatal diagnosis. Molecular diagnosis mainly refers to the detection of genes encoding various structural proteins, enzymes, antigens, antibodies and immunoreactive molecules related to diseases. Polymerase chain reaction (PCR) products with high sensitivity, strong specificity, short diagnostic window period, can be carried out for both qualitative and quantitative detection, which can be widely used in hepatitis, venereal disease, pulmonary infectious diseases, and genetic disease genes of eugenics, tumor, etc. For some diseases, the immune detection window period is about two weeks, but molecular assays can provide important information for early diagnosis and early treatment. The main techniques of molecular diagnosis include nucleic acid molecular hybridization, polymerase chain reaction, biochip technology, etc.

The scope of work in molecular diagnosis includes pathogenic microorganisms, transplantation, genetic diseases, hematological diseases, precision medicine and forensic evidence, such as HBV-DNA quantitative and genotyping, HBV drug-resistant mutation analysis, quantitative and genotyping HIV, HCV RNA, sexually transmitted disease pathogen DNA detection, Human cytomegalovirus, HCMV-DNA quantitative, qualitative and drug-resistant TB-DNA genetic testing, analysis of human leukocyte antigen (HLA) genotyping, HLA antibodies, genetic disease of genetic testing, blood disease related fusion gene screening and quantitative analysis, and human papilloma virus (HPV) typing detection, paternity test, individual identification, bone marrow and peripheral blood karyotype analysis, drug related gene detection, circulating tumor DNA, folic acid receptor detection of circulating tumor cells, detection of genetically related genes of breast cancer, detection of 16 ALL related gene mutations, detection of acute myelocytic leukemia (AML) / myeloproliterative neoplasms (MPN) / myelodysplastic syndrome (MDS) related gene mutations, detection of 58 myeloid gene mutations, etc., providing help for disease prevention, early diagnosis, determination of clinical treatment plans and efficacy judgment.

The laboratory information system can operate without paper, the outpatient department can automatically print the report in time, and the ward can observe the test results in real time, realize the characteristic function of timeliness, accuracy and precision, and serve the clinical diagnosis better. In short, the automated and intelligent laboratory is a vivid portrayal of the development of laboratory medicine in the past 20 years. The efficiency of immune automation in the diagnosis of infectious diseases was further improved, and there were more automatic detection items such as tumor markers, thyroid function, hormones and vitamins. Electrophoresis plays a decisive role in the diagnosis of multiple myeloma in hemoglobin disease. It is particularly worth mentioning that the rapid development of molecular biology in the clinical laboratory, such as hepatitis virus DNA, RNA quantitative detection, HPV typing detection, prenatal diagnosis, and so on. All promote the development and progress of laboratory medicine. Liquid mass spectrometry technology is ascendant. Next-generation sequencing (NGS) technology in prenatal diagnosis, therapeutic drug monitoring, pathogenic microorganism rapid differential diagnosis and drug susceptibility testing, the discovery of drug targets, more and more new technologies, new disease markers, play a greater role in the future. The extensive application of automation and intelligent equipment can reduce the manual labor of laboratory operators, and improve the efficiency and quality of the laboratory, shorten turnaround time (TAT). Meanwhile, laboratory personnel could actively change their roles, reflect their technical ability based on understanding the characteristics of the equipment, and give a strong judgment on the test results.

2.3　Quality control and laboratory management

With the development of science and technology, clinical laboratory testing instruments and methods have made revolutionary progress. It is of great importance to seek a scientific management method to improve the quality of laboratory detection continuously. The International Organization for Standardization (ISO), College of American Pathologist (CAP) and other international standards of the society of the pathologist, come into our field of vision. Health commission defines the definition of medical laboratory for all kinds of samples taken from the body of hematology, biology, chemistry, microbiology, biophysics, immunology, and blood immunology and cytology test. No matter which kinds of standard are chosen to satisfy the basic requirement of laboratory management method, we must establish a comprehensive quality management system first, which includes the core of the technologist of quality assurance, the effective run, and continuous improvement.

The operation of the quality management system should follow the requirements of the quality management system document, and start the operation of the system according to the content specified in the document. Usually, the system should be run for a while, and the system shall be tested through internal supervision and audit to verify whether it has achieved the expected purpose. The medical laboratory should be in daily work, focusing on personnel, testing equipment, sample methods, facilities and environment, testing records, and other key contents, for the supervision and inspection. quality management work may include taking routine inspections, avoiding assay missing, strengthening the system files, carrying out the process management requirements, and so on.

Quality management refers to the organization of quality policy, objectives, job responsibilities, and achievements of all the management functions by quality planning, quality control, quality assurance and quality improvement in the quality system. Chinese National Approval Committee (CNAS), which is responsible for medical laboratory quality and the ability to recognize the special regulations, require the medical laboratory to prove its technical ability of quality management with correct results, including organization and management of the quality system, contract review, document control, laboratory testing, consulting services, external services and supplies, complaint handling, corrective actions and preventive measures, continuous improvement, quality and technical records, internal audit and management review. The technical requirements specify the technical capabilities required for the work of the laboratory, including personnel, facilities and environmental conditions, laboratory equipment, pre-inspection procedures, inspection procedures, quality assurance of inspection procedures, post-inspection procedures, and results reports.

The guidelines for the operation of the quality management system are "the CNAS-CL02

Standards for Accreditation of Quality and Competence of Medical Laboratories" (ISO 15189 : 2007). The quality management system documents are prepared in accordance with the guidelines, for example, the policies, procedures, plans, and standard operating procedures of medical laboratories are documented. The preparation of quality management system documents should follow four principles: systematicness, legality, witness, adaptability. The documents of quality management system of medical laboratory mainly consists of the following contents:

(1) Quality manual: it is the core part of the document structure of the quality management system. It mainly describes the quality management system and organizational structure, clarifies the quality policy and quality objectives, and determines the supporting procedures and responsibilities of each position in the quality management system and their mutual relations.

(2) Procedure document: it is the expansion and specific expression of each element in the quality manual, which should have strong operability and play a connecting role in the system documents. The structure and contents of program files should follow the "5W + 1H" principles: Why, What, Who, When, Where and How.

(3) Standard operating procedure: it is an important part of the quality management system documents, includes the supporting documents and refinement of the procedure documents, and the guidance for the technical personnel in the medical laboratory to carry out specific inspection work.

(4) Record: it is a key element in the quality management system. It provides evidence for the completion and effect of quality activities, and documents for traceability. It is one of the ways to express the results of quality activities in medical laboratories.

The medical laboratory should train all staffs in all relevant contents of the system documents, so that each staff member has a full understanding of the concepts, purposes, methods, principles and standards on which the quality management system is based, and strictly implements them. After the training, strict assessment will be conducted, and the unqualified personnel will be trained and assessed again until the requirements are met. Clear and documented management procedures should be established, including documents preparation, review and approval, management of documents, electronic files management, etc. Comprehensive management of all elements of management requirements and technical requirements could ensure that the requirements of all elements are fully implemented. The difficulty of the medical laboratory quality management system is the process management. The workflow stipulated in the program documents must be strictly implemented to ensure the compliance and effectiveness of the system operation, otherwise the execution of the system documents cannot be guaranteed.

Pre-analysis quality control are actions for the procudues before analysis to guarantee the results true and accurate. Its executive body is different from the one in analysis. This requires full participation, including inspection personnel, clinical physicians, nurses, care staffs and client. Any error or irregularitie can cause the error of the test results. The work of specimens intial processing include: implement SOP files, transmit sample to the lab, ensure the test sample delivery timely and safe. The SOP files make sure what kind of samples would be accepted or refused, in order to ensure the inspection work meet the requirements.

Quality control in the analysis should make sure that the inspection procedures are standardized. A documented analysis procedure system should be established. facilities, environment, equipments, reagents, and standard substances related to the analysis quality should be strictly managed, the measurement value of analysis results should be traced to the source, and the uncertainty of experiments should be comprehensively analyzed. Quality management in analysis mainly includes the management of personnel, sample pretreatment, analysis process, etc.

Post-analysis quality management is completed after the sample testing to make the report accurate, true and correct, thus the results can be directly used in disease diagnosis and treatment. It refers to the total quality control in the process of the final quality control, and improves clinically effective utilization of test data. errors during this process will make the whole management begin well but end badly.

The internal quality audit of medical laboratory quality management system is conducted after the establishment and operation of the quality management system for a period of time, aiming at all elements of the quality management system. The medical laboratory organizes and implements the internal audit by formulating and planning the internal audit plan. The plan should specify the criteria, scope, frequency and method of audit, and should ensure that the entire quality management system is covered. Internal audit mainly reviews the conformity of system documents and accreditation standards, as well as the conformity and effectiveness of the implementation of system documents. Through internal audit of the quality management system, we could timely detect deficiencies in the lab procedures, effectively correct the dificiencies and make a further improvement of the quality management system.

Management review is a formal evaluation of the status and adaptability of the quality management system by the top laboratory manager in terms of the quality policy and objectives. It is a comprehensive inspection of the quality management system. The purpose of the management review is to ensure the stable quality of service in the medical care of patients and to make necessary changes or improvements in a timely manner. The results of the management review are documented, including the objectives for the next phase of the medical laboratory and the corresponding plans and measures, as well as the objectives and corresponding plans and measures for improving the existing or potential problems.

2. 4　Accreditation of clinical laboratory

Experienced from the original manual operation to the automation instrument, we'll go on with the drilling technology, following the international forefront of development, to promote the application and management of laboratory equipment. During these years, great changes take place in laboratory medicine, new technology and equipment will help us to provide accurate clinical service. Constant improving the technological level and management level will promote the modernization of laboratory hardware, make the clinical management normative, reduce the manual operation, and improve work efficiency.

ISO 15189: 2007 was introduced by China laboratory accreditation council for medical laboratories. This kind of accreditation systems infused the technologists with the idea of quality management and approval, thus the clinical laboratory personnel at all levels start to accept international standards of education, and meet the new requirements of determine system. These years, hundreds of clinical laboratories and third-party laboratories have got CNAS recognition. The progress and the change are revolutionary, thought there is no rule for quantity traceability. The establishment of laboratory standardization drives all work of the laboratory, standardizes clinical tests and ensures the quality of tests. It has become the stable cornerstone of In Vitro Diagnostics (IVD) development in the past 20 years with the continuous emergence of new technologies and equipments.

Medical laboratory accreditation is a way of determining a laboratory's ability to engage in a particular test item and calibrate a technique, and provides formal recognition of a medical laboratory's ability to do so. Laboratories are required to attend relevant ability validation protocols as further proof of inspection technology ability. In order to maintain the recognition or accreditation, the laboratory should accept authority on a regular basis after review, to ensure that laboratory continue to conform to the requirements, and check whether the real operating standards are maintained. Approved medical laboratory is usually issued with a recognized institution identification and endorsement of testing and calibration report, showing its approval status. At the same time, the accreditation proves that, the laboratories can meet the requirements of system and provide reliable test results and calibration services. The accreditation of medical laboratory can improve the quality management level and enhance the social trust in the recognized reality. It can continuously improve the reputation of medical laboratory and enhance the trust in patients and medical staff to the laboratory.

The accreditation will help us eliminate the technical barriers in international communication and realize mutual recognition of test results. It is an important reference of the evaluation. Accreditation of technical capacity, professional services and effective staff management of medical laboratories could produce accurate results, realize mutual recognition of test results between hospitals, reduce the cost of repeated tests for patients and ease the burden on patients.

3 *Discussions*

Can you imagine the future development trends of laboratory medicine?

Resources and references

[1] GOPOLANG F, ZULU-MWAMBA F, NSAMA D, et al. Improving laboratory quality and capacity through leadership and management training: lessons from Zambia 2016 – 2018 [J]. Afr J Lab Med, 2021, 10 (1): 1225.

[2] CHERKAOUI A, RENZI G, VIOLLET A, et al. Implementation of the WASPLab™ and first year achievements within a university hospital [J]. Eur J Clin Microbiol Infect Dis. 2020, 39 (8): 1527 – 1534.

[3] HALIASSOS A. Inter-laboratory comparisons and EQA in the mediterranean area [J]. EJIFCC, 2018, 29 (4): 253 – 258.

[4] SCIACOVELLI L, SECCHIERO S, PADOAN A, et al. External quality assessment programs in the context of ISO 15189 accreditation [J]. Clin Chem Lab Med, 2018, 56 (10): 1644 – 1654.

（陈　捷）

CHAPTER 2
CLINICAL CHEMISTRY

1 *Words and phrases*

Mineral　矿物质

Bilirubin　胆红素

Bile acid　胆汁酸

Albumin　白蛋白

Creatinine　肌酐

Uric acid　尿酸

Cystatin C　胱抑素 C

Glucose　葡萄糖

Triglyceride　甘油三酯

Cholesterol　胆固醇

Amylase　淀粉酶

Lipase　脂肪酶

Electrolyte　电解质

Myoglobin　肌红蛋白

Troponin　肌钙蛋白

Ammonia　氨

Lactate　乳酸

Iron　铁

Osmotic pressure　渗透压

Automation　自动化

End-point reaction　终点反应

Colorimetric determination　比色法

Spectrophotometry　分光光度法

Electrochemistry　电化学

Spectrophotometer　分光光度计

Laboratory information system（LIS）　实验室信息系统

Anticoagulant　抗凝剂

Preanalytical error　分析前误差

Hyperlipidemia　高脂血症

Heterogeneous　多相的，异种的

Polydisperse　多分散的

Lipoprotein　脂蛋白

Apolipoprotein　载脂蛋白

Fatty acyl　脂肪酰

Palmitate　棕榈酸酯

Stearate　硬脂酸盐

Oleate　油酸酯

Chylomicron　乳糜微粒

2　*Readings*

2.1　Introduction of clinical chemistry

Clinical chemistry is the discipline consisting of the measurement of biochemical constituents in body fluids, the interpretation of these results in terms of improving the quality of health care, and the pursuit of a biochemical understanding underlying the pathogenesis of disease. The presence of many different types of organic and biochemical constituents in the blood and other body fluids aids in diagnosing various diseases. For instance, if the kidneys are not properly functioning, there will be an inordinate level of toxic wastes in the liquid portion of the blood, either serum or plasma, indicating that the kidneys are not ridding the body of waste products. And in some cases, malfunction of the kidneys may cause the loss of materials such as minerals and proteins that the body should be reabsorbing and using in its metabolism. When certain tissues are damaged, enzymes peculiar to a specific tissue or organ will cause a rise as the cells die, giving a clue about the tissues being damaged. Tests for therapeutic drug levels and drugs of abuse are commonly performed in the clinical laboratory. Common analytes in clinical chemistry laboratory are listed in Table 2 - 1.

Table 2 - 1　Common analytes in clinical chemistry laboratory.

Item combination	Analytes
Liver function test	Bilirubin, Bile acids, Albumin, Total protein, ALT, AST, GGT, ALP
Kidney function test	Creatinine, Urea, Uric acid, Cystatin C

(To be countinued)

(Continued)

Item combination	Analytes
Glucose	Glucose
Lipids	Triglyceride, Cholesterol, LDL-C, HDL-C, apoA, apoB, Lp (a)
Enzymes	LDH, Amylase, Lipase, CHE,
Electrolytes	Na^+, K^+, Cl^-, Ca^{2+}, Mg^{2+}, PO_4^3, HCO_3^-
Blood gases	PCO_2, PO_2, pH
Cardiac markers	Myoglobin, CK-MB, Troponin T and I, NT-proBNP
Others	Ammonia, Lactate , Iron , Osmotic pressure, etc

The examination of a single item in clinical chemistry has its specific clinical significance. For example, the blood glucose level can be used to diagnose diabetes, and increased serum troponin concentration refers to myocardial injury. But sometimes item combinations can better reflect the state of the body or the diagnosis of diseases, such as liver function test, kidney function test, electrolyte testing, lipid testing, and blood gas analysis. Whether the test items are used alone or in combination, and how they are combined, is not determined at will but based on evidence-based medicine.

The earliest biochemical methods used for diagnosing diseases were testing urine for glucose by finding it attractive for ants, boiling and cooling specimens to identify various proteins in body secretions. Nowadays, the chemistry area has become the most automated division of the medical laboratory. Automation is used to assist the laboratory technician in following aspects:

(1) Processing and transport of specimens;

(2) Loading of specimens and reagents into automated analyzers;

(3) Injection, mixing of specimens and reagents;

(4) Calculation and assessment of the results of the tests performed;

(5) Storage of specimens.

Clinical laboratories have many exceptional tests, specimen containers, and handling situations. Nevertheless, if 80% of specimen containers and handling situations can be standardized and automated, the laboratory will achieve a dramatic reduction in its labor usage and costs.

Many small laboratories now have been consolidated into larger, more efficient entities in response to market trends involving cost reduction. In most laboratories, there are one or more large, complex instruments that perform thousands of tests per hour. These instruments are accurate, sensitive, fast, and require that the results be evaluated by the laboratory technicians. Some large medical laboratories may have several sections within the chemistry department that perform only certain specific and specialized assays.

Many aspects of early testing procedures to measure constituents of the blood are still utilized in the modern clinical chemistry laboratory. The original end-point reaction (also called colorimetric determination), where a reaction develops to the greatest extent possible, then ceases, is a methodology fashioned more than a century ago. It is still used, however, it is now performed more effectively. Another method now determines many enzymes and even some nonenzymatic analytes is kinetic reaction, which measures the amount and speed of change occurring in the reagent and sample mixture over a specific period of time. The end-point reaction that required perhaps 30 minutes to reach completion can now be determined by kinetic reaction in only a few seconds. Calculations from basic physics and chemistry principles are also used to provide test results from processes such as spectrophotometry (where a reaction is read by the amount of light transmitted or absorbed in a test reagent) and electrochemistry (chemical reactions that involve an electron transfer).

To provide results from a given sample in an automated system, the sample must first be identified. Following identification, the specimen volume is measured to ensure a sufficient sample is available for all the assays requested.

After making sure a sample is in the proper position, the system will begin the actual procedures. Samples sometimes require pretreatment for certain assays. Reagents and samples will be mixed in the proper proportions and then incubated under certain conditions that may be necessary for the chemical reaction to take place. Some of these conditions include acidity, alkalinity, temperature, and reaction times. The reaction that occurs for the most part in an instrument called a spectrophotometer, will then be analyzed. Results will be calculated, and a valid report will be shown on a visible screen. A printed report can be provided if required. The laboratory information system (LIS) is often interfaced with the chemistry analyzers and results are then automatically transmitted to the physician's office or to the area of the hospital where the patient is hospitalized.

The analytic procedure is fundamental to clinical chemistry. The major steps of the procedure are presented in Table 2 − 2. It begins with the collection of a specimen obtained from a patient; it involves the transport, storage, and pretreatment of the biologic material (eg, blood, urine, cerebrospinal fluid); and it concludes with the measurement steps in producing a laboratory result. The producer and the user have worked in concert over the past years to identify various sources of analytic variations and to eliminate, or at least to minimize these sources.

Table 2-2   Steps involved in requesting, performing, and evaluating a measured quanity.

Steps	
I	The physician requests a test
II	Laboratory personnel performs the assay
	A. Pre-instrumental phase
	(1) Preparation of the patient
	(2) Obtaining the specimen
	(3) Processing the specimen
	(4) Storing the specimen prior to the measuring step
	B. Instrumental phase
	(1) Dispensing the sample into a reaction vessel
	(2) Combining the sample with one or more reagents
	(3) Recording some physical-consequences of the reaction
	(4) Calculating the value of the quantity measured
	C. Post-instrumental phase
	(1) Laboratory and technical staff accept the value as being of good quantity
	(2) The report of the measurement is sent to the requesting physician.
III	D. The physician evaluates the resultant measurement
	(1) The physician assesses whether the measurement could be consistent with other known patient information.
	(2) The physician makes a clinical decision partially based on the reported measurement.

The sample collection process for chemistry is the first and most important step in performing clinical chemistry tests. Subtle changes or errors in collection will invalidate the results of many assays, causing delays in treatment or perhaps administration of the wrong treatment. There are also many different types of specimens required for certain analyses. Some instruments require a particular type of specimen, such as plasma using only heparin as an anticoagulant, although there are several other anticoagulants. Others may accept whole blood, plasma, serum, capillary blood, and other body fluids. When drawing lists are provided for specimen collection, the type of tube and any anticoagulant required will sometimes be specified to avoid errors which may lead to erroneous results from preanalytical error. Arterial blood is used for blood gases but not for other analyses.

Here is a quick review of specimen requirements for chemistry analysis:

(1) Specimens must be properly identified according to standard procedures followed by the facility.

(2) Specimens containing an anticoagulant must be mixed properly to avoid clots.

(3) Hemolysis may release interfering substances.

(4) Lipemia, a high level of fatty materials in the serum or plasma, must be noted for proper interpretation of results, or the specimen should be recollected.

(5) Specimens in tubes with different anticoagulants could not be mixed together.

(6) Timely delivery to the laboratory and proper storage of specimens that will not be analyzed immediately is of great importance.

(7) Sometimes the tube is not completely filled with specimeus, therefore contains less volume than designed for a given amount of anticoagulant. This will result in an improper dilution ratio and will affect results.

(8) Patients being administered intravenous (IV) solutions or who have other implanted devices will require care in the collection of blood. Blood should never be drawn from above an active IV site.

Next, we will take lipid measurement as an example, and discuss the basic biochemistry, clinical significance, and analytical considerations of lipids, with a special emphasis on those involved in cardiovascular disease.

2. 2　Measurement of lipids and lipoproteins

Lipids are ubiquitous in the body tissue and play a vital role in virtually all aspects of life, providing a source of metabolic fuel and energy storage, serving as hormones or precursors of hormones, acting as functional and structural components in cell membranes, and forming insulation to allow nerve conduction or to prevent heat loss.

The causal relationship between increased plasma concentrations of LDL and risk of coronary heart disease (CHD) and the efficacy of LDL lowering to reduce risk was widely acknowledged by the mid-1980s. Awareness of the importance of intervention emphasized the necessity for uniform means of defining hyperlipidemia and CHD risk. Previous practice used arbitrarily defined cutoffs based on prevailing lipid and lipoprotein concentrations in the general population or in local populations of "normal patients". Because of the relative nonspecificity of early chemical methods for cholesterol measurement and the different types of methods then in use, significant biases existed between values obtained in different laboratories, and it was common for "normal" reference intervals to be laboratory specific. This led to the necessity for uniform definitions of hyperlipidemia based on commonly accepted risk-based lipid and lipoprotein cutoffs and the availability of accurate lipid and lipoprotein measurements.

Plasma lipoproteins are heterogeneous and polydisperse macromolecular complexes (Figure 2-1) that vary considerably in size, composition, and function, and consequently present exceptional analytical challenges. Traditionally, lipoprotein concentrations have been expressed in terms of their cholesterol content, because methods developed early on for measuring cholesterol and lipoproteins carried virtually all of the cholesterol circulating in the plasma. This approach simplifies the methods used to determine lipoproteins, because the lipoprotein fractions are only interested in being separated from each other; the other plasma proteins do not have to be removed.

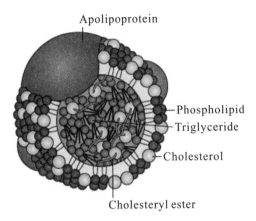

Apolipoprotein

Phospholipid
Triglyceride

Cholesterol

Cholesteryl ester

Figure 2 − 1   The structural components of lipoproteins. (see Appendix Figure 1)

Analytically, cholesterol has a known molecular structure and can be accurately and precisely measured with appropriate chemical or biochemical methods. Triglycerides and the lipoproteins themselves, however, are not unique chemical entities (e. g. , triglycerides consist of many possible fatty acyl groups covalently attached to three positions on a glycerol backbone through ester linkages).

Fatty acyl groups vary in chain length and degree of saturation, leading to a mixture of triglycerides of somewhat different molecular weights. Consequently, triglyceride methods usually measure the glycerol backbone, and triglyceride concentration is then stated only in terms of molar concentration. In the United States, however, lipids have been traditionally expressed in terms of mass concentration (milligrams per deciliter), which is an approximation requiring an assumption about the average molecular weight of the triglyceride mixture. Because palmitate, stearate, and oleate are the major fatty acids in plasma triglycerides and have similar molecular weights, the conversion between molar and mass concentration usually assumes an average triglyceride molecular weight of 885 Da, the molecular weight of tri-oleyl glycerol (olein).

The situation is even more complicated for LDL and HDL. For example, LDL consists of a population of at least seven subparticles varying in size and lipid composition, each containing apo B-100 as the major apolipoprotein component. Thus, LDL has neither a unique molecular weight nor consistent composition of cholesterol or other lipids or proteins. HDL is even more heterogeneous, consisting of at least 12 subclasses, differing in composition, function, and even CHD risk relationships. HDL has been commonly categorized into two major subclasses— HDL_2 and HDL_3 —with the larger HDL_2 fraction showing a stronger inverse association with CHD. Because of these characteristics, the exact concentration and composition of a fraction identified as LDL or HDL may vary, depending on how the fraction is isolated. Once isolated, however, the cholesterol content can be measured accurately. A major consideration, therefore, is to define the lipoproteins in a uniform way to afford a common basis for standardization and the assessment of accuracy without inhibiting the development of new methods or necessitating use of the same methods in all laboratories.

Various technologies have been used to separate and measure plasma lipids, lipoproteins and lipoprotein subfractions, including enzymatic, immunochemical, and chemical precipitation reagents, and physical methods, such as ultracentrifugation, electrophoresis, column chromatography, and so on. As mentioned earlier, the cholesterol content of any particular lipoprotein class can vary somewhat from individual to individual. Moreover, although different methods of lipoprotein separation may produce similar lipoprotein fractions, they usually do not produce identical fractions, giving rise to systematic biases between methods that purport to measure the same component.

Lipid and lipoprotein concentrations vary within individuals when measured on several occasions over time. Sources of variation can be broadly categorized as analytical and physiologic or preanalytical. Analytical variations are inherent in the measurements themselves and arise from sample collection procedures, volume measurements, instrument function, reagent formulations, uncertainty in the assignment of values to calibration materials, and other such factors. Normal physiologic variation occurs independently of analytical error and reflects actual changes in concentration that occur through the course of normal, day-to-day living. Such variations result from factors such as change in posture, which causes the redistribution of water between vascular and nonvascular spaces, thereby changing the concentrations of nondiffusible plasma components. Recent food intake produces transient which increases in plasma triglycerides of 50% or greater, and decreases of up to 10% to 15% in LDL and HDL cholesterol, depending on the fat content of the meal. The shifts result from changes in the lipid composition of lipoproteins that occur as chylomicrons are metabolized. Seasonal changes have also been observed, probably resulting from changes in dietary and exercise patterns throughout the year. Normal physiologic variations tend to occur in both directions, causing lipid or lipoprotein concentrations to vary somewhat about a mean value for a particular patient. Other kinds of physiologic conditions cause changes from the patient's usual steady-state concentrations, for example, acute illness or stress, pregnancy, dietary changes that result in weight loss or gain, changes in saturated fat intake, or the effects of treatment with lipid-lowering medications. In these cases, changes tend to occur in one direction, and they are not considered normal physiologic fluctuations. Lipoprotein concentrations eventually return to original steady-state concentrations when the patient recovers, or a new steady state is achieved.

Because normal physiologic variations occur, it is difficult to evaluate a patient based on a single measurement that applies only to the-current sample. It is more appropriate to consider the patient's usual range of concentrations and his or her average steady-state concentration. From the laboratory's standpoint, the aim is to provide accurate measurements in the particular sample being measured. For this reason, the laboratory is primarily concerned with minimizing analytical error. From the physician's standpoint, however, the goal is to establish the patient's usual range of concentration for purposes of diagnosis and judge the effects of treatment. This aim is affected primarily by physiologic variation, because physiologic variation contributes the larger proportion of the sample-to-sample variation observed in serial samples from the same patient. Some sources of physiologic variation, such as posture during blood sampling, can be controlled; other factors that cannot be controlled, such as pregnancy, should be considered in interpreting laboratory results.

2.3   Analytical variation

Table 2 −3 illustrates the current overall variation of lipid and lipoprotein measurements in more than 100 laboratories participating in an accuracy-based survey conducted by the College of American Pathologists. In this survey, fresh frozen serum is sent to participating laboratories, and the results are compared with the reference method when available. Results from total cholesterol meet the National Cholesterol Education Program (NCEP) error goal for bias and imprecision. The average bias is in the range of − 1.18% to 0.29%, and coefficient of variation (CV) are less than 3%. These numbers represent the totals of within-and among-laboratory components of variation, and suggest that reliable cholesterol measurements can be provided by most clinical laboratories. Similarly, the overall bias and precision of various triglyceride assays are relatively good. For HDL cholesterol (HDL-C), most participants use one of the current direct assays, and the average bias slightly exceed the NCEP-recommended bias of ≤5%; the mean CV of the assays also slightly exceed the ≤4% goal for imprecision. Results for LDL-C are not shown, because freezing of the serum is found to affect the commutability of the material, but the performance of the direct LDL-C assay is comparable with that of the direct HDL-C assay, suggesting the need for improvement. It is important to note that the performance of direct HDL-C and LDL-C assays may not be good in patients with dyslipidemias or other conditions that may affect the specificity of assays for the lipoprotein being measured.

Table 2 −3   Analytical variation of lipid and lipoprotein measurements. *

Analyte	01	02	03
Cholesterol			
Numbers of laboratories	135	135	134
Mean, mg/dL	150.8	179.2	244.9
CV,%	2.1	2.2	1.8
CDC value	152.6	180.0	244.2
Bias,%	− 1.18	− 0.44	0.29

(To be countinued)

(Continued)

HDL – C			
Numbers of laboratories	134	133	135
Mean, mg/dL	31.7	56.6	49.2
CV,%	4.6	3.8	4.7
CDC value	33.9	56.8	49.3
Bias,%	−6.49	−0.35	−0.20
Triglyceride			
Numbers of laboratories	142	141	142
Mean, mg/dL	88.8	204.8	225.7
CV,%	3.2	2.4	2.3
CDC value	91	202.5	223.6
% Bias	−2.42	1.14	0.94

* Bias calculated as: (Test mean-CDC value) / CDC value × 100%

2.4　Physiologic variation

The normal physiologic component of variation is calculated from the total variation of measurements in serial specimens from the same patients, after adjustment for analytical variation. Such estimates differ somewhat from study to study, but after an extensive review of the literature, the NCEP panels concerned with lipid and lipoprotein measurement assume average physiologic CVs (Table 2 - 4). A wide variety of factors contribute to physiologic variations, for example, prior intake of food within a few hours of specimen collection, obesity, diabetes mellitus, nephrosis and pregnancy may result in an increase in chylomicrons. While prolonged fasting, nephrosis and use of cyclosporine will cause an increase in total cholesterol. Physiologic variations observed for cholesterol, HDL cholesterol, and LDL cholesterol are similar. Physiologic variation for triglyceride is considerably higher, because fasting triglyceride concentrations can vary widely within an individual. Because the analytical CVs for these assays are relatively small, it can be calculated that, on average, physiologic variations contribute about 69% to 98% of the overall variance of lipid and lipoprotein concentrations (see Table 2 -4). For this reason, a patient's usual lipid or lipoprotein concentration cannot be reliably established from a single measurement. NCEP guidelines recommend that for cholesterol, the average of measurements in two serial samples obtained at least 1 week apart should be used; two to three serial specimens are recommended, if feasible, for triglyceride and for HDL and LDL cholesterol.

Table 2－4   Physiologic variation in lipid and lipoprotein concentrations in serial specimens from the same individual.

Component	Physiologic variation (CV,%)	Percentage of variance contributed by physiologic variation * (%)
Total cholesterol	6. 5	91
Triglyceride	23. 7	98
HDL cholesterol	7. 5	69
LDL cholesterol	8. 2	81

* Assuming the following analytical *CV*s: total cholesterol, 2% ; triglyceride, 3% ; HDL cholesterol, 5% ; LDL cholesterol, 4%.

3   Discussion

What are the challenges of measuring serum lipids? How to solve them?

Resources and references

[1] RIDLEY J W. Essentials of Clinical Laboratory Science [M]. Boston: Cengage Learning, 2010.

[2] BURTIS C A, ASHWOOD E R. Teitz fundamental of clinical chemistry [M]. 6th ed. St. Louis: W. B. Saunders Company, 2018.

（干　伟）

CHAPTER 3
LABORATORY EXAMINATION OF THYROID GLAND DISORDERS

1 *Words and phrases*

Endocrine hormones　内分泌激素

Anterior pituitary　垂体前叶

Hypothalamus　下丘脑

Hormone homeostasis　激素动态平衡

Secreted in a pulsatile manner　脉冲式分泌

Peripheral hormones feedback　外周激素反馈（调节）

Corticotropin-releasing hormone（CRH）　促肾上腺皮质激素释放激素

Adrenocorticotropin hormone（ACTH）　促肾上腺皮质激素

Somatostatin（SS）　生长抑素

Growth hormone-releasing hormone（GHRH）　生长激素释放激素

Growth hormone（GH）　生长激素

Insulin-like growth factor-1（IGF-1）　类胰岛素样生长因子－1

Gonadotropin-releasing hormone（GnRH）　促性腺激素释放激素

Follicle-stimulating hormone（FSH）　卵泡刺激素

Luteinizing hormone（LH）　黄体生成素

Prolactin（PRL）　催乳素

Thyrotropin-releasing hormone（TRH）　促甲状腺素释放激素

Thyroid-stimulating hormone（TSH）　促甲状腺激素

Thyroid hormones　甲状腺激素

Thyroxine（T_4）　甲状腺素

Free thyroxine（FT_4）　游离甲状腺素

Triiodothyronine（T_3）　三碘甲腺原氨酸

Free triiodothyronine（FT_3）　游离三碘甲腺原氨酸

Thyroid-binding globulin（TBG）　甲状腺结合球蛋白

Thyroid peroxidase antibodies　甲状腺过氧化物酶抗体

Thyrotoxicosis　甲状腺毒症

Hyperthyroidism　甲状腺功能亢进

Subclinical hypothyroidism　亚临床甲状腺功能减退

Subcute thyroiditis　亚急性甲状腺炎

Thyroid nodule　甲状腺结节

Thyroid neoplasm　甲状腺肿瘤

Palpitation　心悸

Hyperhidrosis　多汗

Diffuse goiter　弥漫性甲状腺肿

Nodular goiter　结节性甲状腺肿

Adenoma　腺瘤

2　*Readings*

2.1　Introduction

2.1.1　Endocrine hormones

The anterior pituitary is generally recognized as the "master" of other glands, because together with the hypothalamus, they orchestrate the complex regulation of multiple organs and maintain hormone homeostasis. Hormones are highly potent organic chemicals released by endocrine cells. After being transported by body fluids, hormones play an exciting or inhibitory role in regulating the function of other cells or organs. Endocrinology is a science that studies the hormones secreted by endocrine glands, tissues, and cells in the body. The complete diagnosis of endocrine diseases should include functional diagnosis, localization diagnosis, and etiological diagnosis. Typical cases have particular clinical manifestations, which can provide some clues for disease diagnosis, but early identification of mild or atypical cases is not easy because of the lack of symptoms and/or signs. The determination of endocrine diseases must cooperate with laboratory examinations to correctly identify and treat early. Hypothalamic hormones regulate anterior pituitary tropic hormones to determine target gland secretion. Hypothalamic releasing hormone (RH) can increase the synthesis and secretion of corresponding adenohypophysis hormone, for example, the thyrotropin-releasing hormone can promote the synthesis and secretion of pituitary thyrotropin, hypothalamic inhibitory hormone can inhibit the synthesis and secretion of corresponding pituitary hormone, and prolactin inhibitory hormone can reduce the synthesis and secretion of pituitary prolactin. In turn, peripheral hormones feedback regulates pituitary and hypothalamic hormones (Figure 3 – 1). The hypothalamus secretes corticotropin-releasing hormone (CRH), somatostatin (SS), growth hormone-releasing hormone (GHRH), thyrotropin-releasing hormone (TRH), and gonadotropin-releasing hormone

(GnRH). And there are six major hormones produced by the anterior pituitary, i. e. adrenocorticotropin hormone (ACTH), growth hormone (GH), thyroid-stimulating hormone (TSH), prolactin (PRL), follicle-stimulating hormone (FSH), and luteinizing hormone (LH). All of these hormones are stimulated by specific hypothalamic-releasing factors and secreted in a pulsatile manner.

1. Secretion and mechanism of adrenocortical hormone

ACTH is an important hormone to maintain the normal morphology and function of the adrenal gland. Under the action of hypothalamic corticotropin-releasing hormone (CRH), ACTH is synthesized and secreted by the basophils of the adenohypophysis. Glucocorticoid plays a long negative feedback effect on the hypothalamus and anterior pituitary, and inhibits the secretion of CRH and ACTH. Under physiological conditions, the hypothalamus, pituitary, and adrenal gland are in relative dynamic balance. Lack of ACTH will cause adrenocortical atrophy and decrease of secretory function. ACTH also has a short negative feedback regulation that controls its release. Hypercortisolism, also known Cushing's syndrome (CS), is the most common adrenocortical disease, which is caused by excessive secretion of glucocorticoids (mainly cortisol) by the adrenal cortex for a variety of reasons. According to the etiology, hypercortisolism can be divided into two categories: ACTH-dependent and independent hypercortisolism. The main clinical manifestations are full moon face, concentric obesity, purple skin lines, acne, hypertension, and osteoporosis.

The lesions of the adrenal gland can be hyperplasia, adenoma or cancer. There are more cancers in children. Primary aldosteronism (PA), referred to as proaldehydes, is a disease caused by excessive secretion of aldosterone in the globular zone of the adrenal cortex, resulting in sodium retention and potassium excretion, and the expansion of body fluid volume leads to a series of disorders of secretion and metabolism in the human body. Aldosterone adenoma (aldosterone-producing adenoma, APA) and idiopathic aldosteronism (idiopathic hyperaldosteronism, IHA) are the two most common subtypes, accounting for 70% - 80% and 10% - 20% of primary aldehydes, respectively. Other subtypes include primary adrenocortical hyperplasia (PAH), glucocorticoid-remediable aldosteronism (GRA), aldosterone-secreting adrenocortical carcinoma, familial hyperaldosteronism (FH), ectopic aldosterone secreting adenoma and carcinoma. The main clinical manifestations are hypertension, hypokalemia, changes in muscle strength, abnormal electrocardiogram, and decreased renal concentrating function. Besides, impaired glucose tolerance or diabetes may occur.

2. Secretion and mechanism of growth hormone

Adenohypophysis growth hormone cell (eosinophil) secrete GH. It is a non-glycosylated polypeptide composed of 191 amino acids and the most abundant hormone in the adenohypophysis, accounting for about 50% of adenohypophysis hormones. The daily secretion of the human growth hormone is about $16 \times 20 \mu g /(kg \cdot d)$ in childhood and surges to 20: $38 \mu g /(kg \cdot d)$ in adolescence. Under the influence of exercise, hunger and food, the secretion of human growth hormones can increase $3mg/d$. Although the flow decreases in adults, it lasts until old age. The flow of growth hormone in the human body is pulsed, with an interval of about 3 to 5 hours, and reaches the peak at 1 hour after sleep, and the secretion is more than half of the total secretion in a day. Two neurohormones, i. e. GHRH and SS secreted by the hypothalamus, mainly regulate the secretion of GH. The central nervous system controls the secretion of GHRH adn SS through neurotransmitters such as dopamine, serotonin and norepinephrine.

One of the most important physiological functions of GH is to promote growth and regulate bone metabolism, including the following three points: It stimulates the differentiation and proliferation of chondrocytes at the epiphyseal end to encourage bone growth and increase the length of the bone; It directly stimulates the metabolism of osteoblasts and plays an essential role in maintaining bone mineral content and bone mineral density. Also, GH stimulates chondrocytes to produce insulin-like growth factor-1 (IGF-1), locally to promote chondrocytes proliferation. At the same time, GH stimulates the liver to synthesize IGF-1, acting on the growth plate to make chondrocytes proliferate. So GH promotes bone growth and increases bone length through direct and indirect effects. The second physiological function of GH is to regulate substance metabolism: It encourages protein synthesis and correct negative nitrogen balance. It regulates lipid metabolism, reduces body fat reserve, increases the content of serum fatty acids, and reduces the levels of serum cholesterol and low-density lipoprotein. It can reduce the sensitivity of cells to insulin, reduce the utilization of glucose in peripheral tissues, and increase blood glucose. It plays a vital role in water and mineral metabolism. It can not only retain potash and phosphate in cells but also promote the reabsorption of sodium in renal tubules, resulting in water and sodium retention. Finally, the growth hormone has other physiological functions: increase immunity, stimulate immunoglobulin synthesis and promote the proliferation of macrophages and lymphocytes, accelerate wound healing and stimulate fibroblasts from burn wounds and surgical incisions to synthesize collagen, promote myocardial protein synthesis, increase myocardial contractility, and reduce myocardial oxygen consumption.

3. Secretion and mechanism of prolactin

The anterior pituitary secretes a polypeptide hormone called prolactin. Prolactin in mammals is a single-chain polypeptide composed of 198 amino acids with a relative molecular mass of 21500kDa, containing three disulfide bonds. Most prolactin molecules exist in the circulatory system as monomers. At the same time, in the bloodstream, there are also several kinds of prolactin polymerizing in macromolecules and small-molecules. Prolactin is a single-chain polypeptide hormone secreted by vertebrate adenohypophysis, which has more than 300 different biological functions. Prolactin, as an essential factor for the growth and development of animals, has a direct effect on the division and proliferation of somatic cells. There are two forms of action-circulating hormones and cytokines. When stress reaction occurs, the concentration of prolactin in blood also increases. Like adrenocorticotropin and growth hormone, prolactin is one of the three major hormones secreted by adenohypophysis in stress response. In mammals, prolactin can regulate breast development, promote milk production, initiate and maintain lactation through autocrine and paracrine. Prolactin also plays a role in the periodic growth of hair follicles. Prolactin also has an effect on human ovaries, which stimulates the production of follicular, luteal receptors and permits the biosynthesis of ovarian hormones. Hyperprolactinemia is common in patients with prolactinoma. It can cause ovulation dysfunction, luteal insufficiency, irregular menstruation, milk overflow, and so on. Among them, the primary amenorrhea accounts for 4%, secondary amenorrhea 89%, and menstruation sparse 7%. Dysfunctional uterine bleeding and poor luteal function account for 23% to 77%. Related symptoms include habitual abortion, decreased libido, hirsutism, acne, etc.

4. Secretion and mechanism of sexual hormones

Luteinizing hormone (LH), also known as interstitial cell promoter, is a glycoprotein hormone secreted by basophilic cells of the anterior pituitary, which acts in conjunction with follicle-stimulating hormone to stimulate the ovary to secrete estrogen, progesterone and promote the maturation and discharge of follicles. LH can also support the development of male testicular Leydig cells and promote the secretion of testosterone. FSH is a kind of glycosylated protein hormone synthesized and secreted by the pituitary gland, which regulates a series of physiological processes related to development, growth, puberty, sexual maturation and reproduction. FSH can promote sperm production in male testes and help female ovaries to produce eggs. FSH and LH play an essential role in physiological processes related to reproduction. The two have a synergistic effect of stimulating the development of germ cells and the production and secretion of sex hormones in the ovaries or testis.

5. Secretion and mechanism of thyroid hormones

Thyroid-stimulating hormones (TSH) mainly stimulates the thyroid gland to synthesize and secrete thyroid hormones. The thyroid is one of the endocrine glands in the human body. The increased secretion of thyrotropin will lead to hyperthyroidism, such as hunger, weight loss, fear of heat, sweating, palpitation, handshaking, and sympathetic nervous system excitation, and affect many systems of the whole body. Decreased secretion of thyrotropin will cause hypothyroidism, patients with few words, fatigue, lethargy, anorexia, abdominal distension, constipation and other manifestations, affecting many systems of the whole body. If stimulating thyroid hormone is not secreted enough in childhood, it will affect the growth and intellectual development of children, that is, hypothyroidism. In this chapter, we mainly focus on the disorders of thyroid hormones.

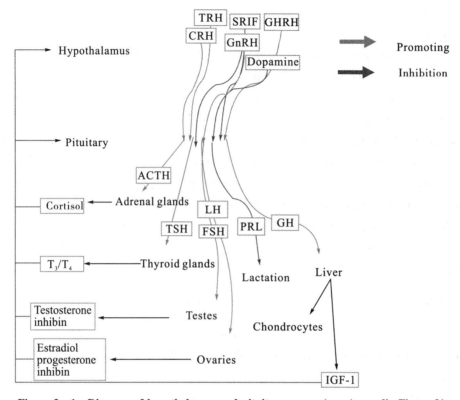

Figure 3 − 1   **Diagram of hypothalamus and pituitary axes.** （see Appendix Figure 2）

CRH, corticotropin-releasing hormone; ACTH, adrenocorticotropin hormone; SRIF, somatostatin, somatotropin release-inhibiting factor; GHRH, growth hormone-releasing hormone; GH, growth hormone; TRH, thyrotropin-releasing hormone; TSH, thyroid-stimulating hormone. T_3, Triodothyroxine; T_4, Thyroxine; GnRH, gonadotropin-releasing hormone; FSH, follicle-stimulating hormone; LH, luteinizing hormone; PRL, prolactin; IGF-1, insulin-like growth factor-1.

2. 2   Laboratory diagnosis of thyroid gland disorders

2. 2. 1   Thyroid hormone

The thyroid is one of the endocrine glands in the human body. The thyroid hormones secreted by the thyroid are essential to the human body, which play a vital role in the metabolism of the human body and maintain the life activities of cells. The more common thyroid diseases are hyperthyroidism and hypothyroidism. In adults, the thyroid gland is the largest endocrine gland, located below the thyroid cartilage of the neck and on both sides of the trachea. Thyroid gland disorders are mainly caused by autoimmune processes which can stimulate the over production of thyroid hormones and lead to hyperthyroidism (thyrotoxicity) or glandular damage and underproduction of thyroid hormones (hypothyroidism). The neoplastic processes can lead to benign nodules or carcinoma of the thyroid gland.

A classic endocrine feedback loop controls the production and secretion of thyroid hormones, including thyroxine (T_4) and triiodothyronine (T_3) (Figure 3 − 1). The thyroid releases large amounts of T_4 and small amounts of T_3, and most T_3 is produced by the deiodination of T_4 in peripheral tissues. In circulation, most T_4 and T_3 are bound to carrier proteins (thyroid-binding globulin, TBG, transthyretin (only bind T_4) and albumin). The small parts of T_3 and T_4 are in a free state. open state and binding state of thyroid hormones maintain balance. Only FT_3 and FT_4 can play a role in peripheral tissues. The functions of thyroid hormones include maintaining growth and development, promoting metabolism, nervous system and cardiovascular effects, etc. In chronic liver disease, nephrosis and systemic illness, total T_4 and T_3 levels decrease and free levels are normal. On the contrary, the increased total T_4 and T_3 levels, and normal free levels suggested for increasing carrier proteins, such as pregnancy, hepatitis, inherited disorders.

2. 2. 2   Detection techniques

The detection methods of TSH include radioimmunoassay (RIA), enzyme-linked immunosorbent assay (ELISA) and electrochemiluminescence immunoassay (ECLIA), etc. The functional sensitivity of the first generation TSH is 1. 0 mIU/L to 2. 0 mIU/L, represented by RIA, which could only distinguish normal thyroid function from hypothyroidism, but could not distinguish hyperthyroidism from normal thyroid function. The functional sensitivity of the second generation TSH is 0. 1 mIU/L to 0. 2 mIU/L, also known as sensitive TSH (sTSH), represented by IRMA, which can distinguish TSH levels from normal and mild hyperthyroidism. However, it is not able to test the TSH levels below the functional sensitive after hyperthyroidism treatment. The third generation TSH assay, also known as ultrasensitive TSH (uTSH), is represented by immunochemiluminescence and time-resolved immunofluorescence. The functional sensitivity of uTSH is 0. 01 mIU/L, and the specificity is high. In patients with normal hypothalamus-pituitary gland, the determination of TSH can replace the TRH excitation test to evaluate the inhibition of pituitary gland.

In serum, T_4 is all secreted by the thyroid, so it is an excellent index to reflect the state of thyroid function. T_3 is the active form of thyroid hormone. The sum of binding state and free state is total T_4 (TT_4) and total T_3 (TT_3). The detection methods include RIA and ECLIA. The FT_3 and FT_4 are not affected by TBG and directly reflect the functional status of the thyroid. The detection methods include balanced dialysis, radioimmunoadsorption, chemiluminescence, and electrochemiluminescence immunoassay.

TSH receptor autoantibody (TRAb) is an autoantibody produced in patients with autoimmune thyroid disease. They are polyclonal antibodies, including thyroid-stimulating antibody (TSAb), thyroid functions inhibitory antibody (TFIAb), and thyroid growth immunoglobulin (TGI), and they bind to thyroid receptors to produce different biological effects. The detection methods include RIA, bioanalysis, ELISA and so on.

The anti-thyroglobulin antibody (TgAb) and anti-thyroid peroxidase antibody (TPOAb) are two primary thyroid autoimmune antibodies, derived from lymphocytes in the thyroid. They are autoantibodies against thyroglobulin, thyroid peroxidase, and other antigens. As a sign of immune dysfunction, most of them exist in patients with autoimmune thyroid disease (AITD). The detection methods include radioimmunoadsorption, electrochemiluminescence immunoassay and so on.

2.2.3　Thyroid dysfunction

1. Laboratory examination

At present, serum TSH is the most commonly used, reliable, and sensitive test to evaluate thyroid function. TSH is the most sensitive index for the diagnosis of hypothyroidism. The value of TSH and thyroid hormones is as follows: $TSH > FT_4 > TT_4 > FT_3 > TT_3$. The coincidence rate of early diagnosis and prediction of recurrence of hyperthyroidism is $TSH > FT_3 > FT_4 > TT_3 > TT_4$. At present, the determination of TSH can replace the TRH excitation test and the T_3 inhibition test. TSH is affected by sleep and emotion, and has a circadian rhythm, so a single result should not judge it. The process of sample collection also affects the test results.

Serum TT_3 and TT_4 can directly reflect the thyroid function, but their levels are affected by the concentration of thyroid-binding globulin in the circulation.

Serum FT_3 and FT_4 exist in a free state in the bloodstream, which represents the level of thyroid hormones in the tissue, which is consistent with the metabolic state of the body and is not affected by thyroid-binding globulin. It is used to judge the state of thyroid function and monitor the changes of disease during treatment. In general, the changes of FT_3 and FT_4 are consistent with those of TT_3 and TT_4. FT_3, FT_4, TT_3, and TT_4 increase in hyperthyroidism, while FT_3, FT_4, TT_3 and TT_4 decrease in hypothyroidism. FT_4 is a sensitive index for the diagnosis of hypothyroidism, better than that of FT_3. In the treatment of hyperthyroidism, FT_3 is a useful index for observing the curative effect, better than that of FT_4.

Serum Tg is a marker to predict tumor residue and recurrence. Determination of serum Tg content is helpful in judging prognosis and monitoring the effectiveness of treatment. During the clinical follow-up of patients with differentiated thyroid cancer, it was found that the determination of Tg content had high sensitivity and specificity in the diagnosis of recurrence or metastasis of differentiated thyroid cancer. But Tg negative can not rule out recurrence or metastasis. In subacute thyroiditis, the level of Tg increased significantly, and Tg returned to normal quickly after the inflammation was controlled. Tg levels may continue to grow in some patients with painless thyroiditis. Due to the increased level of Tg in nodular goiter, rare malignant tumors cannot be screened by Tg in benign sarcoidosis.

The epidemiological survey of TgAb and TPOAb showed that the positive rates of TgAb and TPOAb in the population were 3% – 11.5% and 10% – 15%, respectively. The positive rates of TgAb and TPOAb increased with age, and the positive rate of females was significantly higher than that of males. The positive rates of TgAb and TPOAb in patients with Hashimoto's thyroiditis were 80% - 90% and 90% - 100%, respectively. The positive rates of patients with Graves disease were 50% - 70% and 50% - 80%, respectively.

rT_3 is mainly used to observe the peripheral metabolism of thyroid hormone. The increase of TT_4 and rT_3 is in hyperthyroidism and the decrease of TT_4 and rT_3 in hypothyroidism. The reduction of TT_3 and/or TT_4 and the abnormal growth of rT_3 support the diagnosis of the non-thyroid morbid syndrome, which may be caused by the decline of peripheral 5' deiodinase activity.

The hypothalamus synthesizes TRH and the function of TRH is to promote pituitary synthesis and secretion of TSH. The fluctuation of TSH concentration after intravenous injection of TRH can observe the response of pituitary to TSH and understand the reserve capacity of TSH. This examination is a basic method to know the function of the hypothalamus-pituitary-thyroid axis.

2. Laboratory diagnostic criteria

Secondary hyperthyroidism: the serum TSH increases or maintains normal, while the levels of TT_4, FT_4, TT_3, and FT_3 increase.

Primary hypothyroidism: serum TSH increases, while the levels of TT_4, FT_4, TT_3 and FT_3 decrease.

Secondary hypothyroidism: serum TSH decreases or maintains normal, while the levels of TT_4, FT_4, TT_3 and FT_3 decrease.

Subclinical hyperthyroidism: the serum TSH decreases, while the levels of TT_4, FT_4, TT_3 and FT_3 are normal.

Subclinical hypothyroidism: the serum TSH increases, while TT_4, FT_4, TT_3 and FT_3 are normal.

2.2.4   Hypothyroidism

In almost all varieties of hypothyroidism, the levels of FT_4 decrease. Elevated serum TSH levels are sensitive to primary hypothyroidism, but not found in secondary hypothyroidism. About 90% of hypothyroidism patients caused by autoimmune diseases are positive for TPO antibodies. Evaluation of thyroidism are summarized in Figure 3 - 2. At the same time, laboratory tests show increased levels of cholesterol, creatine phosphokinase, and anemia. The ECG displays bradycardia, flatted or inverted T waves and low amplitude QRS complexes.

1. Laboratory examination

TSH is the most sensitive index for the diagnosis of hypothyroidism. When TSH increases,

FT_3, FT_4, TPOAb, and TgAb, should be tested to confirm the early diagnosis of subclinical hypothyroidism or autoimmune thyroid disease (AITD). TSH is also the main screening index of neonatal hypothyroidism.

Serum FT_3 and FT_4 in patients with hypothyroidism generally decrease, mild hypothyroidism, the initial stage of hypothyroidism mainly decreases FT_4, while subclinical hypothyroidism FT_3, FT_4 are normal.

TgAb and TPOAb are used to distinguish autoimmune thyroid diseases from non-autoimmune thyroid diseases. The degree of thyroid damage is different in different types of autoimmune thyroid diseases so that the titer of TgAb and TPOAb can judge it. The general rule of titer is Hashimoto's thyroiditis > Graves disease > non-autoimmune thyroid disease. The presence of TgAb and TPOAb in patients with subclinical hypothyroidism indicates that the disease is more likely to develop into clinical hypothyroidism because of AITD, and the presence of high titers of these two antibodies in GD patients indicates that spontaneous hypothyroidism is more likely to occur.

The levels of serum TT_3 and TT_4 in patients with severe hypothyroidism are lower than those in patients with severe hypothyroidism, but TT_3 in patients with mild hypothyroidism does not necessarily decrease, and TT_4 is more sensitive than TT_3.

TRH stimulation test shows the level of thyroid hormone decreased, and the response to TRH increased in patients with primary hypothyroidism. In patients with secondary hypothyroidism, if the lesion is delayed in the hypothalamus, and the injury is in the pituitary, there is no response. TRH stimulation test can also be used for follow-up observation of hypothyroidism patients.

2. Laboratory diagnostic criteria

The diagnostic criteria of adult hypothyroidism and subclinical hypothyroidism are mostly based on the laboratory criteria issued by the American Society of Thyroid Diseases (1990). However, the American Society of Clinical Endocrinology, the Royal College of Physicians, and the European Society of thyroid Diseases have different diagnostic criteria. The principle is that TSH is the first-line indicator. If TSH increases, the possibility of primary hypothyroidism should be considered. However, a single determination of serum TSH can not be diagnosed as hypothyroidism, FT_3, FT_4, and other indexes can be added if necessary, and attention should be paid to the critical TSH value. There is no clinical manifestation of hypothyroidism, but the increase of TSH, with or without the decrease of FT_4, can generally be diagnosed as subclinical hypothyroidism. The diagnostic criteria of pituitary hypothyroidism are TSH decreaseding or maintaining normal, and FT_4, FT_3 decreasing. The diagnosis of hypothalamic hypothyroidism depends on the TRH stimulation test. The standard of screening neonatal hypothyroidism is different from that of clinical hypothyroidism, and the critical value of serum TSH is generally set as 20 mIU/L.

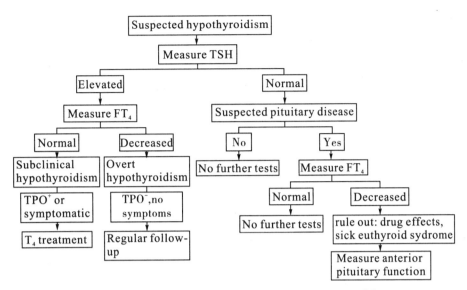

Figure 3 − 2   Diagnosis and treatment path for hypothyroidism.

TPOAb $^+$, thyroid peroxidase antibodies present; TPOAb $^-$, without thyroid peroxidase antibodies; FT$_4$, free thyroxine; TSH, thyroid-stimulating hormones.

2. 2. 5   Hyperthyroidism

Serum TSH is a sensitive biomarker of hyperthyroidism (thyrotoxicosis) caused by thyroiditis, Graves disease, autonomous thyroid nodules, and exogenous levothyroxine treatment. Accompanying with the abnormalities of liver enzymes, bilirubin, and ferritin. Thyroid radioiodine uptake provides a clue for etiological diagnosis for hyperthyroidism: high uptake rate indicates Graves disease and nodular disease, low uptake rate indicates iodine excess, thyroid destruction and extrathyroidal sources. In subacute thyroiditis, the ESR evaluated. The summary of the evaluation of hyperthyroidism is shown in Figure 3 − 3.

1. Laboratory examination

The coincidence rate of thyrotropin (TSH) in the diagnosis and prediction of recurrence of early hyperthyroidism is in the following order: TSH > FT$_3$ > FT$_4$ > TT$_3$ > TT$_4$.

In the diagnosis and treatment of hyperthyroidism, the sensitivity of serum FT$_3$ is better than that of FT$_4$ and TT$_4$. FT$_4$ is of high value in the diagnosis and treatment of hypothyroidism.

The concentration of rT$_3$ in serum maintains a certain proportion with TT$_3$ and TT$_4$, exceptionally consistents with the evolution of T$_4$, which can be used as an index to understand thyroid function. In the early stage of hyperthyroidism or recurrent hyperthyroidism, only rT$_3$ increased. In severe malnutrition or some systemic diseases, rT$_3$ increases dramatically, while TT$_3$ decreases substantially, which is an essential index for the diagnosis of the non-thyroid morbid syndrome.

The levels of TRAb: (1) To diagnose untreated GD patients, the sensitivity of the TSAb test (85% - 100%) was higher than that of the TBII test (75% - 96%). (2) To determine the efficacy of antithyroid drugs in the treatment of GD and predict recurrence: after the use of antithyroid drugs in patients with hyperthyroidism, the titer of TRAb decreases, indicating that the treatment was effective. At present, it is considered that if TRAb continues to be positive after antithyroid drug treatment in GD, and it has a specific predictive value for indicating recurrence. (3) To diagnose Graves ophthalmopathy (GO), it is closely related to GD hyperthyroidism. The titer of TSAb can reflect the degree of ocular lesions in patients with GO. TSAb in patients with GO is significantly higher than that in patients with non-GO GD, and severe patients often have a high titer of TSAb. (4) Prediction of thyroid dysfunction in newborns and lactating infants: when pregnant women suffer from GD, the mother is usually positive for TRAb and can enter the fetus through the placenta, causing neonatal hyperthyroidism. TRAb is best detected at three months of pregnancy, and the positive rate of TRAb will decrease in the middle and third trimester of pregnancy. TRAb can be secreted from breast milk and thyroid function is normal, but breast-feeding in TRAb-positive women can also lead to hyperthyroidism in infants. The TRAb of neonatal hyperthyroidism originates from the mother and is not produced by itself. With the extension of time, TRAb can be degraded by itself, and the symptoms of hyperthyroidism will be gradually relieved, so without treatment, most of them can be relieved spontaneously at 1 - 3 months after birth, with no recurrence. If the newborn has GD, its TRAb may be persistently positive, and the symptoms can not be relieved by itself. (5) To detect the tendency of GD in relatives of GD patients: because of the hereditary tendency of GD, if the relatives of GD patients were positive for TRAb or TSAb, they might develop into obvious GD in the future. 50% - 90% of GO patients with TgAb and TPOAb have different titers of TgAb and TPOAb. Persistently high titers of TgAb and TPOAb often indicate that spontaneous hypothyroidism is more likely to occur in the future.

TRH stimulation test diagnosis of hyperthyroidism: typical hyperthyroidism patients with elevated thyroid hormone levels inhibit the pituitary response to TRH, so hyperthyroidism patients have no answer to the TRH stimulation test. However, with the application of sTSH and uTSH, this test has been rarely used in the diagnosis of typical hyperthyroidism.

Prediction of remission and recurrence of hyperthyroidism: after antithyroid drugs were used to treat hyperthyroidism, the response to TRH indicated that the function of hypothalamus-pituitary-thyroid axis could be restored, and the recurrence of hyperthyroidism was less, so it is seldom used at present.

2. Laboratory diagnostic criteria

Hyperthyroidism with elevated serum FT_3, FT_4 or TT_3, TT_4 and decreased TSH; only increased FT_3 or TT_3 but normal FT_4 or TT_4 could be considered as type T_3 hyperthyroidism;

only increased FT_4 or TT_4 and normal FT_3 or TT_3 could be regarded as type T_4 hyperthyroidism; and decreased TSH, normal FT_3 and FT_4 were consistent with the diagnosis of subclinical hyperthyroidism.

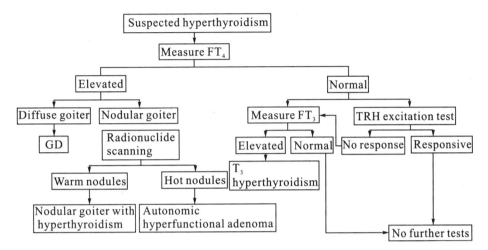

Figure 3 – 3   Etiology and differential diagnosis of hyperthyroidism.

GD, Graves disease; FT_4, free thyroxine; T_3, triiodothyronine; FT_3, free triiodothyronine; TRH, thyrotropin-releasing hormone.

3   *Discussion*

Clinical features: Female, 48 years old.

Chief complaint: palpitations, hyperhidrosis, weight loss for six months, photophobia, and tears for one month.

Six months ago, there was palpitation and hyperhidrosis, and the weight decreased about 15kg in about half a month, and photophobia, tears, and double vision occurred one month ago.

Physical examination: BP is 138/80 mmHg, and heart rate is 90 beats per minute. The bilateral upper eyelid contracture, bulbar conjunctiva hyperemia, edema, bulbar protrusion, cannot be completely closed, inward movement disorder, and upward, lower, and outer movement is right — the bilateral thyroid enlargement of degree Ⅱ, soft quality, no tenderness, and unpalpable nodules. The superior bilateral thyroid can hear a murmur. There were no positive signs in the heart, lung and abdomen, and no mucinous edema in both lower extremities.

Supplementary examination: TSH 0.02 mIU/L, FT_3 10.5 pmol/L, FT_4 50 pmol/L, rT_3 1.0 nmol/L, TPOAb 20 IU/mL, TRAb 65 IU/L. Thyroid ultrasound showed diffuse, symmetrical, and homogeneous enlargement of the thyroid gland. Double orbital CT showed a double anterior process. Several extraocular muscle showed thickening.

Case analysis: The patient was a middle-aged woman with typical clinical manifestations of thyrotoxicosis, including visible eye signs, bilateral thyroid enlargement of degree II, and vascular murmur. Thyroid ultrasound showed "thyroid diffusely enlarged", and the elevation of FT_3, FT_4, and rT_3 suggested hyperthyroidism. Because TSH was suppressed, it was primary (thyroid) hyperthyroidism. The biorbital CT was recommended the changes of Graves ophthalmopathy. The elevated TRAb supported Graves disease.

Diagnosis: Hyperthyroidism, Graves disease, Graves ophthalmopathy grade IV.

Resources and references

[1] MELMED S, JAMESON J L. Harrison's principles of internal medicine: anterior pituitary: physiology of pituitary hormones [M]. 19th ed. New York: McGraw-Hill, 2018.

[2] Jameson J L, Mandel S J, Weetman A P. Harrison's principles of internal medicine: disorders of the thyroid gland [M]. 20th ed. New York: McGraw-Hill , 2019.

[3] TAYLOR P N, ZHANG L, LEE R W J, et al. New insights into the pathogenesis and nonsurgical management of Graves orbitopathy [J]. Nat Rev Endocrinol, 2020, 16 (2): 104 - 116.

[4] BIONDI B, CAPPOLA A R, COOPER D S. Subclinical hypothyroidism: a review [J]. JAMA, 2019, 322 (2): 153 - 160.

[5] CITTERIO C E, TARGOVNIK H M, ARVAN P. The role of thyroglobulin in thyroid hormonogenesis [J]. Nat Rev Endocrinol, 2019, 15 (6): 323 - 338.

[6] JONKLAAS J, RAZVI S. Reference intervals in the diagnosis of thyroid dysfunction: treating patients not numbers [J]. Lancet Diabetes Endocrinol, 2019, 7 (6): 473 - 483.

[7] CHAKER L, CAPPOLA A R, MOOIJAART S P. Clinical aspects of thyroid function during ageing [J]. Lancet Diabetes Endocrinol, 2018, 6 (9): 733 - 742.

[8] BIONDI B, COOPER D S. Subclinical hyperthyroidism [J]. N Engl J Med, 2018, 378 (25): 2411 - 2419.

[9] TAYLOR P N, ALBRECHT D, SCHOLZ A, et al. Global epidemiology of hyperthyroidism and hypothyroidism [J]. Nat Rev Endocrinol, 2018, 14 (5): 301 - 316.

[10] CHAKER L, BIANCO AC, JONKLAAS J, et al. Hypothyroidism [J]. Lancet, 2017, 390 (10101): 1550 - 1562.

[11] CHANSON P, SALENAVE S. Diagnosis and treatment of pituitary adenomas: a review [J]. JAMA, 2017, 317 (5): 516 - 524.

[12] VAN DEN BELD A W, KAUFMAN J M, ZILLIKENS M C, et al. The physiology of endocrine systems with ageing [J]. Lancet Diabetes Endocrinol, 2018, 6 (8): 647 - 658.

（何　詠）

CHAPTER 4

MOLECULAR GENETICS

1 *Words and phrases*

Genetics　遗传学

Mutation　突变

Genome　基因组

Genotype　基因型

Chromosome　染色体

Polymerase chain reaction（PCR）　聚合酶链反应

Denaturation　变性

Primer annealing　引物退火

Elongation　延伸

Fluorescence in situ hybridization（FISH）　荧光原位杂交

Restrict fragment length polymorphisms（RFLPs）　限制性酶切片断长度多态性

Nucleic acid sequence-based amplification（NASBA）　核酸序列依赖性扩增

Transcription-mediated amplification（TMA）　转录介导的扩增技术

Multiplex ligation-dependent probe amplification（MLPA）　多重连接探针扩增技术

Comparative genomic hybridization（CGH）　比较基因组杂交

Immunoblotting　免疫印迹

Karyotyping　核型分析

Insertion　插入

Deletion　缺失

Duplication　重复

Inversion　倒位

Translocation　易位

Dideoxy chain termination（Sanger）sequencing　双脱氧链终止(Sanger)测序

DNA rearrangement　DNA 重排

Next-generation sequencing（NGS）　二代测序

Linkage analysis　连锁分析

Circulating nucleotide acids　循环核酸

Amplification refractory mutation system（ARMS）　扩增阻滞突变系统

Digital PCR（dPCR）　数字 PCR

Autosomal dominant（AD）　常染色体显性遗传

Autosomal recessive（AR）　常染色体隐性遗传

X-linked inheritance　X 连锁遗传

Pedigree　系谱

Proband　先证者

Sib　同胞

Sibship　同胞群

Mendel's laws of inheritance　孟德尔遗传定律

Malformation　畸形；变形

Trinucleotide repeat　三核苷酸重复

Homozygous　纯合子的

Heterozygous　杂合子的

Huntington's disease　亨廷顿舞蹈症

Duchenne muscular dystrophy（DMD）　杜氏肌营养不良

Spinal muscular atrophy（SMA）　脊髓性肌萎缩

Amyotrophic Lateral Sclerosis（ALS）　肌萎缩侧索硬化

Polyglutamine　多聚谷氨酰胺

Prodrome　前驱症状

Dementia　痴呆

Dysarthria　构音障碍

2　Readings

2.1　Introduction

2.1.1　Human chromosome

A fundamental feature of human biology is that each generation reproduces by combining haploid gametes containing 23 chromosomes, resulting from independent assortment and recombination of homologous chromosomes. Over the past three decades, remarkable progress has been made in our understanding of the structure and function of genes and chromosomes. It is well known that the DNA double helix highly is agglutinated to form chromosomes. Each human cell contains a complete set of 23 pairs, 46 chromosomes. During cell division （mitosis）, the chromosomes duplicate so that new cells produced contain the same number and kinds of chromosomes as the original. Among them, 22 pairs are autosomes and the other pair are sex chromosomes. The sex chromosomes, which determine the sex of offspring, differ from the other 22 pairs. The female has two similar chromosomes called X chromosome while the male has two different chromosomes, one X chromosome, and one Y chromosome. (Figure 4 - 1, Figure 4 - 2)

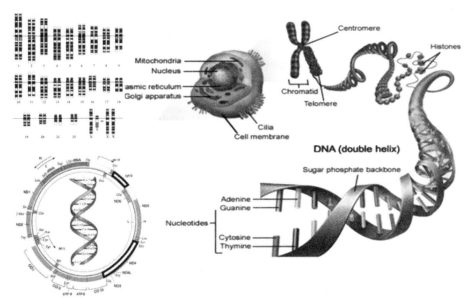

Figure 4 - 1   The DNA strands are highly condensed to form chromosomes.

(Science Learning Hub-Pokapū Akoranga Pūtaiao. Retrieved from www. sciencelearn. org. nz)

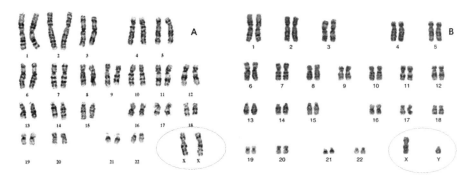

Figure 4 - 2   Normal human chromosome. (A: Female; B: male).

Every nucleated cell in the body carries its copy of the human genome, which contains, by current estimates, 25,000 genes. Each gene has a precise position or locus. A gene map is the map of the chromosomal location of the genes and characteristics of each species and each individuals within a species.

DNA is a polymeric nucleic acid macromolecule composed of three types of a five-carbon deoxyribose sugar, a nitrogen-containing base, and one of the four phosphates: adenine, cytosine, guanine, and thymine. The double helical structure of DNA was first described by

James Watson and Francis Crick in 1953. The helical structure resembles a right-handed spiral staircase in which its two polynucleotide chains run in the opposite direction, and hold together by hydrogen bonds between pairs of bases: A paired with T, and G with C. The genetic information is encoded in the sequence of C's, A's, G's, and T's. Thus, the anatomical structure of DNA carries the chemical information and allows the exact transmission of genetic information from one cell to its daughter cells and from one generation to the next.

Each human chromosome consists of a single, continuous DNA double helix. The genome is packaged as chromatin, in which genomic DNA is complexed with several classes of chromosomal proteins. When a cell divides, its genome condenses to appear as microscopically visible chromosomes.

The flow of genetic information is referred to as the central dogma of molecular biology, which is, genomic DNA directs the synthesis and sequence of RNA, RNA directs the synthesis and sequence of polypeptides. Also, some specific proteins are involved in the synthesis and metabolism of DNA and RNA.

2.1.2   Tools of molecular genetics—the basic

One of the principal aims of medical genetics is to characterize mutations that leads to genetic disease, to understand how these mutations affect health, and to improve diagnosis and management. Here are some basic tools for examination of the RNA or DNA from a particular gene that can be used to distinguish a particular disease.

1. Polymerase chain reaction

The polymerase chain reaction (PCR) has become the most powerful molecular genetic technique available and resulted in a Nobel Prize (Mullis, 1987). PCR essentially duplicates the in vivo replication of DNA in vitro with the same result: one copy of double-stranded DNA becoming two copies. The components of PCR, including DNA template, short oligonucleotide primer, nucleotides, polymerase, and buffers, are subjected to an amplification program which consists of a specified number of cycles with multiple repetitions of denaturation, primer annealing, and chain elongation by heat-stable polymerase. It involves the use of primers that flank the molecular genetic region of interest (typically up to 1000 base pairs are amplified) and is done on a thermal cycler. It is much more sensitive than the Southern or Northern blot and amplifies DNA (or RNA by reverse transcriptase PCR). PCR has been used for the detection of point mutations and chromosomal translocations, DNA fingerprinting, and infectious disease identification.

2. Restricted fragment length polymorphisms (RFLP) typing

RFLP was first described in 1980s and is observed as differences in size and number of fragments generated by restriction enzyme digestion of DNA. The first step of RFLP is to construct a restriction enzyme map of the DNA region under investigation, and polymorphisms are detected by observing fragment numbers and sizes different from those expected from the reference restriction map. Once the restriction map is known, the number and sizes of the restriction fragments of a test DNA region cut with a restriction enzyme are compared with expected fragments based on the restriction map. DNA is cut with restriction enzyme and resolved by gel electrophoresis, blotted to a membrane. Probes to specific regions of DNA containing potential RFLPs are then hybridized to DNA on the membrane to determine the size of the resulting bands. Fragment sizes may vary as a result of changes in the nucleotide sequence in or between the recognition sites of a restriction enzyme. Every genotype will yield a descriptive band pattern due to recombination and random assortment, and each person has a unique set of RFLPs, half inherited maternally and half paternally. Nucleotide changes may also destroy, change, or create restriction enzyme sites, altering the number of fragments.

3. Karyotyping

A karyotype is the complete set of chromosomes in a cell. Karyotyping is the direct observation of metaphase chromosome structure by arranging metaphase chromosomes based on size. It requires collecting living cells and growing them in culture for 48 to 72 hours in the laboratory. Cell division is stimulated by the addition of mitogen and dividing cells are arrested in metaphase. The 23 pairs of chromosomes can then be assembled into a karyotype according to their size and centromere placement. Aneuploidy affecting several chromosomes or a single chromosome can be observed by karyotyping and other chromosomal mutations, such as translocations (including balanced, unbalanced, and Robert translocation), deletions, insertions, inversions and ring chromosome can also be observed.

4. Fluorescence in situ hybridization

Fluorescence in situ hybridization (FISH) is a method widely used to detect protein and RNA as well as DNA structures in place in the cell, or a situ. The development of fluorescence in situ hybridization allows detection of specific nucleic acid sequences in metaphase chromosomes and, potentially, interphase nuclei. FISH offers a more rapid assay with higher resolution and flexibility than karyotyping. For FISH cytogenetic analysis, fixed cells are exposed to a probe. The probe will hybridize, or bind, to its complementary sequences in the cellular DNA. This method is useful in identifying chromosomal abnormalities but requires knowledge of the abnormality of interest as probes are designed to be complementary to a particular chromosome or chromosomal locus so that the image under the microscope will correlate with the state of that chromosome or locus. There are several types of probes such as signal, multiple, dual fusion, break-apart, and centromeric probes.

5. Dideoxy chain termination (Sanger) sequencing

The Sanger sequencing method is a modification of the DNA replication process involving synthesis of a complementary DNA template using natural 2'-deoxynucleotides (dNTPs) and termination of synthesis using 2', 3'-dideoxynucleotides (ddNTPs) by DNA polymerase. Modified ddNTPs derivatives are added and lack the hydroxyl group found on 3' ribose carbon of deoxynucleotides which will stop upon the incorporation of ddNTP into the growing DNA chain and terminate the chain synthesis. For detection of the products of the sequencing reaction, the primer may be attached covalently at the 5' end to a fluorescent dye-labeled nucleotide. Balanced appropriately, competition between synthesis and termination processes results in the generation of a set of nested fragments, which differ in nucleoside monophosphate units. The nested fragments are then separated by their size using high-resolution gel electrophoresis and as these dye-labeled fragments pass through the detection region, fluorophores are excited by the laser in the DNA sequencer, producing fluorescence emissions of four different colors. The determination of the color is the underlying method for assigning a base call, and the order of the fluorescent fragments reveals the DNA sequence. The ratio of dNTP/ddNTP in the sequencing reaction is critical for the generation of the readable sequence, and hence the distribution of lengths of terminated chains. If the ddNTP concentration is too low, infrequent or no termination will occur and if the ddNTP concentration is too high, polymerization will terminate too frequently early along with the template.

6. Multiplex ligation-dependent probe amplification

Multiplex ligation-dependent probe amplification (MLPA), first reported in 2002, is a relatively simple and robust multiplex PCR method for detecting chromosomal DNA copy number changes in multiple targets. For a short sequence of target DNA, two adjacent probes are designed that contain the forward and reverse primer sequence, respectively. In addition, one of the probes contains a stuffer sequence of which the length can be varied in function of the experiment. The probes are hybridized against the target DNA and subsequently ligated. Only if ligation happens, a functional PCR strand appears, so that amplification only happens if target DNA is present in the sample. The amount of PCR product is proportional to the amount of target DNA present in the sample, making the technique suitable for quantitative measurements. Multiple probe pairs are pooled and amplified with the same primer pair so that the technique does not suffer from the typical limitations of multiplex PCR.

2.1.3 Tools of molecular genetics—the advanced

Molecular technology continues to evolve rapidly. In the future, new molecular technology will enable the use of smaller samples, decrease turnaround time, and allow for automation to avoid the intense labor that initially made molecular pathology difficult for routine clinical use. It would appear that the most effective laboratory organizational structure in terms of cost, quality, and expertise to handle this rapidly expanding technology is to structure molecular pathology as a core area of the pathology laboratories, with the maintenance of a dynamic interaction with other areas of the laboratory.

1. Next-generation sequencing

Next-generation sequencing (NGS) represents an entirely new principle of sequencing technology following Sanger (first generation) sequencing. Next-generation sequencing is designed to sequence large numbers of templates simultaneously, yielding not just one, but hundreds of thousands of sequences in a run within a few hours. This means that NGS is based on the principle of "sequencing-by-synthesis" and the complementary integration of a nucleotide during chain prolongation is directly monitored by the sequencing machine. With the advent of NGS, throughput exploded to up to > 1 tera bases (= 1012 or, in other words, 1000 billion bases) and this enormous improvement has been achieved by massively parallel sequencing. The goal of NGS is to achieve the sequence of the human genome for a minimal cost, known as $1000 genome, making genetic studies a routine component of both clinical analysis and research. Three platforms for massively parallel DNA sequencing read production are in reasonably widespread use at present: the Roche/454 FLX, the Illumina/Solexa Genome Analyzer, and the Applied Biosystems SOLiDTM System. NGS is a powerful tool to detect variants within the genome of any given individual. With genome sequencing, about 4 million variants per individual can be detected, whereas exome sequencing (covering mainly the 1 % protein-coding part of the genome) results in about 20, 000 variants. NGS is not only useful in large extended families, where linkage information provides information about the disease locus, but may also be applied to detect disease-causing de novo mutations in sporadic patients. Finding a disease-causing variant among these many alterations mirrors the proverbial search for the needle in the haystack.

2. Digital PCR (ddPCR)

Digital PCR is a new method of nucleic acid detection and quantitative analysis, which can be used as an alternative to traditional real-time quantitative PCR to achieve absolute quantitative and rare allele detection. Digital PCR works by dividing DNA or cDNA samples into many separate, parallel PCR reactions, some of which contain the target molecule (positive) and others (negative). A single molecule can be amplified a million times or more. During amplification, TaqMan chemical reagents and dye-labeled probes can be used to detect specific sequences of targets. When there is no target sequence, there is no signal accumulation. After PCR analysis, the negative reaction fragment is used to generate an absolute count of the target molecule in the sample, without the need for standard or internal standards. As there is no need to rely on references or standards, the accuracy of digital PCR can be improved by using more

PCR replicators and having high tolerance to inhibitors. Digital PCR can analyze complex mixtures and linear detection of small multiple changes.

3. Comparative genomic hybridization

Comparative genomichybridization (CGH) is a technique based on the competitive in situ hybridization of differentially labeled DNA from endometriosis and normal endometrial tissue to human metaphase spreads. Microarrays are a new technique that allows a large number of different genetic sequences to be arrayed on a slide which can then be used to identify specific sequences in an unknown mix of either DNA or RNA. This technique requires the development of DNA synthetic techniques and microprocessor-controlled robotics for array design and it has been used extensively in cell biology. CGH can scan the whole genome with high reproducibility, higher resolution, and throughput, and with no cell culture and it can be independent from microscope. CGH can also detect CNVs at a submicroscopic level and deletions of single genes as causative of features of larger microdeletion syndromes and it allows for a genotype-first approach rather than a phenotype-first approach for new syndrome identification.

2. 2　Laboratory diagnosis of genetic disorders

According to the existing form of a pathogenic gene or chromosome change, human genetic diseases are generally divided into three types: single-gene diseases, polygenic genetic diseases, and chromosomal diseases. Multifactorial genetic disease, known as polygenic disease, involves many genes, as the main gene is difficult to be identified, so it cannot be effectively diagnosed by molecular biology. Single-gene traits caused by a mutation in genes in the nuclear genome are often called Mendel's laws of inheritance. The single-gene diseases known so far are listed in Mendelian Inheritance in Man (OMIM) and are available on the internet through the National Library of Medicine with more than 3917 diseases caused by mutations in 1990 genes.

　　Single-gene traits caused by a mutation in genes in the nuclear genome are often called a single locus. A person is called homozygous if he/she has a pair of identical alleles and heterozygous when the alleles are different. Single-gene disorders are characterized by their patterns of transmission in families. The first step to establish the pattern of transmission is to obtain information about the family history of the patient and to summarize the details in the form of pedigree-a graphical family tree with standard symbols. The member through whom a family with a genetic disorder is first brought to the geneticist is the proband no matter affected or not. Brothers and sisters are called sibs, and a family of sibs forms a sibship.

　　The patterns of inheritance of single-gene disorder in families depend chiefly on two factors: (1) whether the phenotype is dominant (expressed with only one mutation allele while the other chromosome has a wild-type allele) or recessive (only expressed when both chromosomes carry mutant alleles) and (2) whether the chromosomal location of the gene locus is on an autosome (chromosome 1 – 22) or on a sex chromosome (chromosome X or Y). Also, it is necessary to distinguish the physical location of genes on the sex chromosomes (X or Y synteny) and genes that show X-linked or Y-linked inheritance.

An important component of medical genetics is identifying and characterizing the genotypes responsible for particular disease phenotypes. Genetic heterogeneity maybe result from different mutations at the same locus (allelic heterogeneity), mutations at different loci (locus heterogeneity), or both. Distinct phenotypes inherited in different families can result from different mutant alleles in the same gene. Most of the recessive disorders described to date are due to mutations that reduce or eliminate the function of the gene product, so-called loss-of-function mutations. In contrast, a phenotype expressed in both homozygotes and heterozygotes for a mutant allele is inherited as a dominant.

2. 2. 1   Autosomal inheritance

1. Characteristics of autosomal recessive inheritance

An autosomal recessive phenotype, if appears in more than one member of a kindred, typically is seen only in the sibship of the proband, not in parents, off-springs, or other relatives. Parents of an affected child are asymptomatic carriers of mutant alleles and may in some cases be consanguineous especially when the gene responsible for the condition is rare in the population. For most autosomal recessive diseases, there is no difference in affection between males and females.

2. Characteristics of autosomal dominant inheritance

Common subtypes include (1) complete dominance; (2) incomplete dominance; (3) irregular dominance; (4) common dominance; (5) delayed dominance; and (6) from the dominant sex.

The phenotype usually appears in every generation, each affected person having an affected parent. However, there are some exceptions: (1) cases originating from fresh mutations in a gamete of phenotypically normal parents; and (2) cases in which the disorder is not expressed or expressed only subtly in a person who has inherited the responsible mutant allele.

Any child of an affected parent has a 50% risk of inheriting the trait. Although this is true for most families, there maybe exceptions as statistically, each family member is the result of an "independent event", wide deviation from the expected 1 : 1 may occur by chance in a single family. Phenotypically normal family members do not transmit the phenotype to their children but the failure of penetrance or subtle expression is not included in this rule. Like autosomal recessive phenotype, males and females are equally likely to transmit the phenotype to children of either sex. A significant proportion of isolated cases are due to new mutations.

The less the fitness is, the greater the new mutation might be.

2.2.2 X-linked inheritance

Approximately 1100 genes are though located on the X-linked chromosome, of which approximately 40% are presently known to be associated with disease phenotypes. As males have one X chromosome but females have two, there are two possible genotypes in males and three in females in mutant allele at an X-linked locus. So, the use of terms dominant and recessive is somewhat different in X-linked conditions than for autosomal disorders.

1. Characteristics of X-linked recessive Inheritance

The incidence of disease in males is much higher than in females. Heterozygous females are usually unaffected, but some may express the disease with variable severity as determined by the pattern of X inactivation. The gene responsible for the disease is transmitted from an affected man through all his daughters and any of his daughters' sons has a 50% chance of inheriting it but will never be transmitted directly from father to son. The mutant allele maybe transmitted through a series of carrier females; if so, the affected males in kindred are related through females. A significant proportion of isolated cases are due to new mutations.

2. Characteristics of X-linked dominant inheritance

Affected males with normal mates have no affected sons and no normal daughters. Since the pathogenic gene is dominant and located on the X chromosome, only one of the pathogenic genes XA occurring in both men (XAY) and women (XAXa) can cause the disease. Both male and female offspring of female carriers have a 50% risk for inheriting the phenotype. The pedigree pattern is similar to what is seen with autosomal dominant inheritance. But unlike autosomal dominant inheritance, female patients can pass the disease-causing genes to both their children and daughters with equal opportunities and men can only pass on the gene to their daughters, not their sons. Affected females are approximately twice as common as affected males, but affected typically have milder, although variable, expression of the phenotype.

2.2.3 Diagnostic pathways for genetic diseases (Take HD for example)

The main mutation types of single-gene diseases include point mutation, insertion, deletion, inversion, etc. The selection of laboratory diagnostic techniques depends on the characteristic mutation types of specific diseases.

1. The characteristic of HD disease

An example of autosomal dominant disease is Huntington's disease. Huntington's disease (HD), a neurodegenerative disorder, is caused by a heterozygous expanded trinucleotide repeat $(CAG)_n$, encoding glutamine, in the gene encoding Huntingtin (HTT) on chromosome 4p16.

The incidence of HD varies greatly from country to country and region to region, with a low incidence in Asia of about 0.1 to 2.0 per 100,000. The diagnosis of HD depends on positive family history, characteristic clinical manifestations, and the detection of 36 or more CAG trinucleotide repeats in the Huntington protein-coding gene (HTT gene). The pathogenic mutations in HTT can be detected in almost 100% of HD patients. Huntington's disease is an autosomal dominant disorder. The mutant huntingtin protein in HD results from an expanded CAG repeat leading to an expanded polyglutamine strand at the N terminus and a putative toxic gain of function. Neuropathologic studies show neuronal inclusions containing aggregates of polyglutamines. When the number of CAG repeats reaches 41 or more, the disease is fully penetrant. Incomplete penetrance can occur with 36 to 40 repeats (Figure 4 - 3). The number of repeats accounts for approximately 60% of the variation in age at onset, with the remainder determined by modifying genes and environment. The increasing CAG trinucleotide repeat sequence (or polyglutamine) in exon 1 leads to changes in the structure and biochemical properties of the huntington protein, which finally causes the disease. The classic signs of Huntington's disease are progressive chorea, rigidity, and dementia. A characteristic atrophy of the caudate nucleus is seen radio graphically. The natural course of Huntington's disease includes early symptoms, prodrome and apparent symptom, and the average age of onset is about 45 years. About two thirds of the patients have first show neurological symptoms, and the symptoms of chorea gradually become apparent as the disease progresses, with difficulty in voluntary activities and even complete dependence on others for help, as well as increased vocal and swallowing difficulties and intermittent aggressive behavior. The median survival time after onset was 15 - 18 years, and the mean age of death was 54 - 55 years old.

As an autosomal dominant disease, children with HD parents have a chance of 50% for developing the disease. The paternal genetic dominants show earlier onset, while maternal genetic dominants onset later. Like other more l-glutamine (CAG) repeat disease, Huntington's disease presents an early genetic phenomenon, earlier onset from generation to generation with heavier symptoms. Typically, Adult HD patients have 40 - 55 CAG repeats, while adolescent HD patients have more than 60 CAG repeats, usually inherited from their fathers. Molecular genetic test results of HTT gene can provide supportive diagnosis and differentiation basis for clinic.

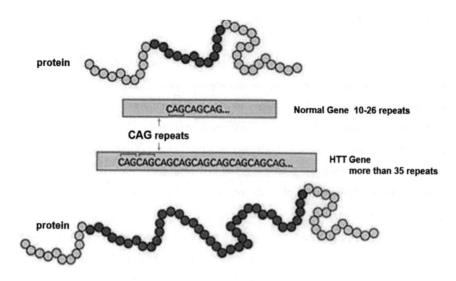

Figure 4 − 3   HDD gene and protein.

2. Related examinations for HD disease

CAG repeats in pathogenic gene (HTT): the accuracy of fluorescent labeled PCR combined with capillary electrophoresis can be accurate to 1bp, so fragment length can be accurately detected to determine the number of CAG repeats on the related pathogenic gene (HTT). (see Figure 4 − 4)

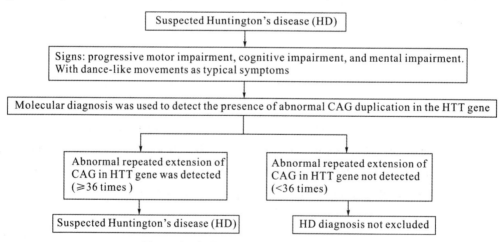

Figure 4 − 4   Laboratory diagnosts of HD.

Triplet repeat-primed PCR with capillary electrophoresis: formerly known as triplet primer PCR, it is suitable for the detection of ultra-long repeat sequences in a variety of genetic dynamic mutant diseases, and can detect abnormal amplification with more than 100 repeats. The amplified products are then analyzed by capillary electrophoresis for fragments analysis, which actually detect a group of small fragments with 1 CAG repetition difference. The length of the repeat sequence could not be accurately obtained, and only the length of the pathogenic repeat sequence could be known.

Normal PCR plus long distance PCR can detect abnormal amplification with more than 100 repetitions. Current capillary electrophoresis equipment cannot carry out electrophoresis of more than 1000bp, so the product of long-distance PCR still cannot accurately obtain the length of repeated sequences, therefore it is generally not preferred.

3 *Discussion*

History: Patient, male, 38 years old. The patient has suffered from head shaking, mouth twitching and lip twitching for 5 years, as well as personality changes, irritability and memory loss. One year ago, the symptoms aggravated with involuntary movement of limbs and trunk and abnormal aggravation of mental behavior.

Physical examination: intermittent facial twitching, dancing movements of limbs, difficulty in autonomous movement, dysarthria, impaired memory and numeracy, impaired comprehension and judgment.

Laboratory examination: CAG duplication times in the HTT gene was analyzed, and the results should abnormal expansion of CAG repeats was detected as 42 times.

Analysis: The patient showed typical clinical symptoms as dance-like motor, cognitive and mental disorders and had abnormal extension of CAG repeats in the HTT gene as 42 times while in the normal population was no more than 35 times.

All three aspects: clinical symptom, physical examination, and laboratory examination suggested that the patients should be diagnosed as Huntington's disease.

In this chapter, after discussing common and advanced technology for molecular genetics in passage one, the typical patterns of transmission of single-gene disorder are discussed in detail in passage two: the emphasis is on the molecular and genetic mechanisms by which mutations in genes results in recessive, dominant, X-linked and mitochondrial inheritance patterns. In these disease, an accurate determination of family pedigree is an important part of the work-up of every patient. Not only is a determination of the inheritance pattern important for asking a diagnosis in the proband, but it also identifies other individuals in the family who may be at risk and in need of evaluation and counseling. However, diseases such as myocardial infarction, cancer, mental ill, diabetes, and Alzheimer disease with high morbidity and mortality, are thought to result from complex interaction between a number of genetic and environmental factors and therefore add even more complexity to individual disease risk and the pattern of disease inheritance.

Q1: What are the three steps of a standard PCR cycle?

A1: The three step of PCR cycle are: denaturation, annealing and extension.

Q2: Please list the common next-generation sequencing systems

A2: 454 sequencing, SOLID system, and Illumina genome analyzer.

Q3: Given the pedigree below, what is /are the most likely inheritance pattern (s); possible but less likely inheritance pattern (s); and incompatible inheritance pattern (s)?

Inheritance pattern(s) includes autosomal recessive(AR), autosomal dominant(AD), X-linked recessive(XR), X-linked dominant, and mitochondrial.

Please give the reason for your choices.

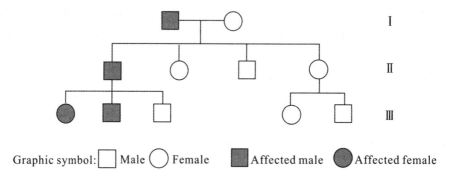

Graphic symbol: ☐ Male ◯ Female ■ Affected male ● Affected female

A3: AD is most likely, as the disease transmitted from generation to generation and from male to male, and both male and female are affected. AR and XR are possible but less likely. AR would require both spouses of the affected individuals are carriers. XR would require two spouses be carrier in generation I and II. X-linked dominant, and mitochondrial are incompatible as there is male to male transmission.

Q4: Case discussion

A 6 years old boy was related to mild development delay, decreased strength and endurance with difficulty in climbing stairs and physical activities. His parents, two brothers and one sister were all healthy. The boy had proximal weakness and his serum creatine kinase level was 50 - 100 higher than normal. The result of muscle biopsy showed marked variation of muscle fiber size, fiber necrosis, fat and connective tissue proliferation. The boy was given a provisional diagnosis of Duchenne muscular dystrophy (DMD) and tested the deletion of the dystrophin gene and found to have a deletion of exons 45 through 48. Subsequent testing showed his mother to be a carrier. The family was therefor seek for genetic consultant.

(1) What's the risk of the parents for having another affected son?

(2) Dose the daughter have the risk of been affected and what does the risk depends on?

(3) What other disease may associated with DMD and what other physical examination should they take?

References and resources

[1] FEERO W G, GUTTMACHER A E, COLLINS F S. Genetic medicine-an updated primer [J]. New Engl J Med, 2010, 362 (21): 2001 – 2011.

[2] BUCKINGHAM L. Molecular diagnostics [M]. 2nd ed. Philadelphia: F. A. Davis Company, 2012.

[3] ROBERT L N, RODERICK R M, HUNTINGTON F W, et. al. Thompson &thompson genetics in medicine [M]. 8th ed. Philadelphia: Elsevier, 2016.

[4] GEOFFREY S G, HUNTINGTON F W. Genomic and personalized medicine [M]. 2nd ed. New York: Elsevier, 2012.

[5] LODISH H, BERK A, MATSUDAIA P, et. al. Molecular cell biology [M]. 7th ed. New York: WH Freeman, 2012.

[6] MOORE K L, PERSAUD T V N, TORCHIA M G. The developing human: clinically oriented embryology [M]. 9th ed. Philadelphia: W. B. Saunders, 2013.

[7] GARDNER R J M, SUTHERLAND G, SHAFFER L, et. al. Chromosome abnormalities and genetic counseling [M]. 4th ed. Oxford: Oxford University Press, 2012.

[8] JORDAN J M G, HASTINGS RJ, MOORE S. ISCN 2020: an international system for human cytogenomic nomenclature (2020) (cytogenetic and genome research) [M]. Basel: Karger, 2020.

[9] TRASK B. Human cytogenetics: 46 chromosome, 46 years and counting [J]. Nature Rev Genet, 2002, 3 (10): 769 – 778.

[10] BAXTER R, VILAIN R. Translocational genetics for diagnosis of human disorders of sex development [J]. Annu Rev Genomics Hum Genet, 2013, 14: 371 – 392.

[11] BAI Y Q. Medical English Reading I [M]. Beijing: People's Medical Publishing House, 2005.

[12] BENNETT R L, FRENCH K S, RESTA R G, et. al. Standardized human pedigree nomenclature: update and assessment of the recommendations of the national society of genetic counselors [J]. J Genet Counsel, 2008, 17 (5): 424 – 433.

[13] PYERITZ R E, KORF B R, GRODY W W, et. al. Emery and Rimoin's essential medical genetics [M]. 7th ed. Oxford: Academic Press, 2018.

[14] SCRIVER C R, BEAUDET A L, SLY W S, et. al. The metabolic and molecular bases of inherited disease [M]. 8th ed. New York: McGraw-Hill, 2000.

[15] BORDELON YM. Clinical neurogenetics: Huntington disease [J]. Neurol clin, 2013, 31 (4): 1085 – 1094.

[16] CARON N C, WRIGHT G E B, WARBY S C, et. al. Huntington disease [J/OL]. GeneReviews, [2020 – 7 – 11] http://www. Ncbi. nlm. nih. gov/books /NBK1305/.

（叶远馨）

CHAPTER 5
TRANSFUSION MEDICINE

1 *Words and phrases*

Blood group　血型

Lipid bilayer　磷脂双分子层

International Society of Blood Transfusion（ISBT）　国际输血协会

Association for the Advancement of Blood & Biotherapies（AABB）
血液与生物治疗促进协会

Intravascular hemolysis　血管内溶血

Extravascular hemolysis　血管外溶血

Renal failure　肾功能衰竭

N-acetylgalactosamine　N－乙酰半乳糖胺

Galactose　半乳糖

Fucose　岩藻糖

Fucosyltransferase　岩藻糖基转移酶

Oligosaccharides　低聚糖

Glycoprotein　糖蛋白

Glycolipid　糖脂

Salivary gland　唾液腺

Epitope　表位

Bombay phenotype　孟买型

Para-Bombay phenotype　类孟买型

Hemolytic disease of the fetus and newborn（HDFN）　胎儿和新生儿溶血病

Hemolytic transfusion reaction（HTR）　溶血性输血反应

Autoimmune and drug-induced hemolytic anemia（AIHA）
自身免疫性及药物诱导性溶血性贫血

Hemagglutination　红细胞凝集反应

Mononuclear phagocyte system　单核吞噬细胞系统

Antiglobulin test　抗球蛋白试验

Direct antiglobulin test（DAT）　直接抗球蛋白试验

Indirect antiglobulin test（IAT）　间接抗球蛋白试验

Enzymes technique　酶技术

Sialic acid　唾液酸

Bromelin　菠萝蛋白酶

Ficin　无花果酶

Papain　木瓜酶

Trypsin　胰蛋白酶

Chymotrypsin　糜蛋白酶

Neuraminidase　神经氨酸酶

Elution technique　放散技术

Disseminated intravascular coagulation（DIC）　弥散性血管内凝血

Transfusion-associated circulatory overload（TACO）　输血相关循环超负荷

Transfusion-related acute lung injury（TRALI）　输血相关急性肺损伤

Transfusion-associated dyspnea（TAD）　输血相关的呼吸困难

Allergic reaction　过敏反应

Transfusion-associated hypotension　输血相关性低血压

Febrile non-hemolytic transfusion reaction（FNHTR）　发热性非溶血性输血反应

Acute hemolytic transfusion reaction（AHTR）　急性溶血性输血反应

Delayed hemolytic transfusion reaction（DHTR）　迟发性溶血性输血反应

Delayed serologic transfusion reaction（DSTR）　输血相关性迟发性血清反应

Transfusion-associated graft vs. host disease（TA-GVHD）
输血相关性移植物抗宿主病

Post-transfusion purpura（PTP）　输血后紫癜

Transfusion-transmitted infection（TTI）　输血传播感染

Antihistamine　抗组胺制剂

Diphenhydramine　苯海拉明

2　*Readings*

2.1　Introduction

2.1.1　History

Blood had been taken as the mysterious resourc of vitality and courage which could cure many ailments in ancient times. It has been thought that the first transfusion happened in 1492 by Pope Innocent Ⅷ who infused three young man's blood to cure his disease but failed. From

1500 to 1800, many researchers attempted to transfuse between animals, and then animal to human being. In 1901, Karl Landsteiner, an Austrian scholar, discovered the ABO blood groups and explained the serious reactions that occured in humans as a result of incompatible transfusion. His work in the early 20th century won him a Nobel Prize in 1930.

Transfusion medicine has developed for centuries, and now is one of the medical-technical disciplines that makes many modern medical therapies possible. This chapter includes blood groups, techniques used in transfusion medicine, and transfusion reactions.

2.1.2   Blood groups

Many proteins, which anchor or cross the red blood cell (RBC) membrane, carry different blood group antigens. The International Society of Blood Transfusion (ISBT) currently recognizes more than 360 antigen specificities, which belong to 43 blood group systems, 5 collections, 17 low incidence antigens and 7 high incidence antigens. The blood group system represents either a single gene or a cluster of closely linked homologous genes. The ABO and Rh systems are the best-known and clinically most important blood group systems. The remaining systems can be checked on ISBT website (http://www.isbtweb.org/working-parties/red-cell-immunogenetics-and-blood-group-terminology/).

2.1.3   ABO and H systems

The ABO system consists of four antigens, A, B, AB, and A1, which are the indirect products of the *A* and *B* alleles of the *ABO* gene. A third allele, *O*, produces no antigen and is recessive to *A* and *B*. There are four phenotypes: A, B, AB, and O. The A phenotype results from the genotypes *A/A* or *A/O*, B phenotype from *B/B* or *B/O*, AB from *A/B*, and O from *O/O*. The famous Landsteiner's rule states that individuals lacking A or B antigen from their red cells have the corresponding antibody in their plasma. In fact, violations of Landsteiner's rule in adults are rare. As histo-blood-group antigens, ABO antigens can be found not only on red cells, platelets, and many circulating proteins in blood but also on many tissues, including those of the endothelium, heart, kidney, pancreas, and lung. ABO-incompatible blood transfusion can be associated with acute intravascular hemolysis, renal failure, and death. Likewise, transplantation of ABO-incompatible organs is associated with acute humoral rejection. To avoid the dire clinical consequences associated with ABO incompatibilities, ABO typing and ABO compatibility testing remain the foundation of pre-transfusion testing and an important component of testing before transplantation.

The H system has only one antigen, H, which is defined by the terminal disaccharide fucose $\alpha 1 \rightarrow 2$ galactose. Two different fucosyltransferase (FUT) are capable of synthesizing H antigen: H gene (FUT_1) and secretor gene (FUT_2). FUT_1 specifically fucosylates Type 2 chain oligosaccharides on red cell glycoproteins and glycolipids to form Type 2 chain H. In contrast, FUT_2 recognizes Type 1 chain precursors to form Type 1 chain H and Le[b] antigens in secretions. Secretion of Type 1 chain ABH antigens in saliva and other fluids requires a functional FUT_2 gene. FUT_2 is not expressed in red cells but salivary glands, gastrointestinal tissues, and genitourinary tissues. Type 1 chain ABH antigen presenting on red cells is passively adsorbed from circulating glycolipid antigen present in plasma.

H antigen is the precursor to both A and B antigens and is expressed on all red cells except the rare Bombay phenotype. In group A individuals, an N-acetylgalactosamine is added, in an $\alpha 1 \rightarrow 3$ linkage, to the subterminal galactose of the H antigen to form A antigen. In group B individuals, an $\alpha 1 \rightarrow 3$ galactose is added to the same subterminal galactose to form B antigen. In group AB individuals, both A and B structures are synthesized. In group O individuals, neither A nor B antigens are synthesized as a result of a mutation in the ABO gene. So the amount of H antigen on red cells depends on an individual's ABO type and is represented thus: $O > A_2 > B > A_1 > A_1 B$.

2.1.4 RH system

Another important blood group system is Rh system which is the most complex blood group system containing at least 55 different antigens, encoded by two Rh genes—RHD and $RHCE$. RHD accounts for many epitopes of D, and $RHCE$ codes both the Cc and Ee polypeptides with four alleles at this locus: $RHCE$, $RHCe$, $RHcE$, and $RHce$. Rh-negative individuals lack the RHD gene and thus that polypeptide. This explains why the d antigen was never found.

Most D-positive red cell phenotypes have conventional RhD protein. However, more than 200 different RHD alleles have been reported. These alleles encode proteins with amino acid changes that can cause numerous variations in the expression of D. The red cells with altered D expression can be encountered in routine transfusion practice. About 1% to 2% individuals of European ethnicity carry RHD alleles that encode altered D antigens, and the incidence in individuals of African ethnicity is higher. There are three familiar categories of altered D: weak D, partial D and DEL.

The weak D phenotype was defined as red cell with a reduced amount of D antigen. For performing no or weak ($\leq 2 +$) reactivity in initial testing, it required indirect antigloblin test (IAT) for detection. It is estimated that the weak D phenotype expressed approximately 0.2% to 1% in Caucasians and 0.01% in Asians. In North London, the prevalence of weak D phenotypes is estimated to be 0.3% to 1.7% in blood donors.

The partial D is the phenotype that has an amino acid substitution in at least one of the extracellular or RBC membrane surface loops resulting in the loss of D epitopes and also generating new antigens. There are 119 partial D types listed by the Rhesus database (http://www.rhesusbase.info/). DVI, one of the most common Partial D categories types, is most likely to be associated with the formation of anti-D.

DEL variant antigens cannot be detected by routine serologic methods, but can be characterized by careful adsorption-elution studies or RHD genotyping. About 10% to 30% of

D-negative people of Asian ancestry are DEL phenotype which is much less common in individuals of European ancestry (0.027%).

To prevent anti-D immunization of recipients, the Association for the Advancement of Blood & Biotherapies (AABB) Standards for Blood Banks and Transfusion Services require donor blood to be tested by a method designed to detect weak expression of D. When the D type of a patient is determined, a weak D test is not necessary except to assess the red cells of an infant whose mother is at risk of D immunization.

2.1.5   Techniques used in transfusion medicine

Routine blood grouping still relies primarily on hemagglutination between antigens and antibodies that are read and interpreted either manually or by automated means. Antiglobulin methods and enzyme technology are introduced as routine methods for the detection of antigen-antibody reactions and play a part in the discovery and expansion of knowledge of blood group systems in general. Since these advances, non-routine methods become available for specialist investigations and as research tools, such as flow cytometry and analysis of antigens at the molecular level.

2.1.6   Tube testing for ABO grouping

ABO grouping requires both antigen typing of red cells for A and B antigen (red cell grouping or forward typing) and screening of serum or plasma for the presence of anti-A and anti-B isoagglutinin (serum grouping or reverse typing). Both red cell and serum or plasma grouping are required for donors and patients because each grouping serves as a check on the other.

Steps:

a. Prepare 5 clean tubes and label them with: anti-A, anti-B, A_1 cell, B cell and O cell.

b. Prepare 2% ~5% suspension of the red cells to be tested.

c. Operate by taking the steps in the table below. (Table 5 - 1)

Table 5 - 1   Operating steps of tube testing.

Step	Action
Testing red cells	
1	Place 1 drop of anti-A in a clean, labeled test tube.
2	Place 1 drop of anti-B in a separate, clean, labeled tube.
3	To each tube, add 1 drop of a 2% to 5% suspension of the red cells to be tested.
4	Gently mix the contents of the tubes; then centrifuge for the calibrated spin time.
5	Read, interpret, and record the test results.

(To be countinued)

(Continued)

Step	Action
Testing serum or plasma	
1	Add 2 or 3 drops each of serum or plasma to two clean, labeled test tubes.
2	Add 1 drop of A_1 reagent red cells to the tube labeled A_1.
3	Add 1 drop of B reagent red cells to the tube labeled B.
4	Gently mix the contents of the tubes; then centrifuge for the calibrated spin time.
5	Examine the serum overlying the red cell buttons for evidence of hemolysis. Gently resuspend the cell buttons, and examine them for agglutination.
6	Read, interpret, and record test results.

d. Interpretation of the tests is given in the table below. (Table 5 − 2)

Table 5 − 2 Interpretation.

Red cell group		Serum group			Interpretation
anti − A	anti − B	A_1	B	O	
+	−	−	+	−	A
−	+	+	−	−	B
−	−	+	+	−	O
+	+	−	−	−	AB
−	−	+	+	+	Bombay/Antiboby existing

2.1.7 The antiglobulin test

The antiglobulin test, which is also referred to as anti-human globulin (AHG) test and Coombs test, is based on the principle that antihuman globulins obtained from immunized nonhuman species binding to human globulins such as IgG or complement, either free in serum or attached to antigens on red blood cells (RBCs). The principle of using anti-human globulins was first described by Moreschi in 1908, but it was not until 1945 that Robin Coombs introduced it to clinical medicine initially as a method to demonstrate RBC agglutination in the presence of what was then thought to be an "incomplete" or "blocking" antibody. Now it is an essential testing methodology for transfusion medicine.

There are two forms of the AHG test, the direct antiglobulin test (DAT) and the indirect antiglobulin test (IAT).

The DAT reflects in vivo antibody sensitization of erythrocytes. Erythrocytes are washed three times to remove any unbound antibodies, and AHG reagent (usual anti-IgG with or without anti-C3d) is then added. If the erythrocytes are coated with IgG antibodies or complement, the AHG reagent will cause them to agglutinate. Clinical conditions that can result in DAT positive are in the following:

- Hemolytic transfusion reactions (HTRs).
- Hemolytic disease of the fetus and newborn (HDFN).
- Autoimmune and drug-induced hemolytic anemia (AIHA).

The IAT is used to detect the presence of IgG antibodies in serum. Reagent erythrocytes are incubated in the serum that potentially contains antibodies. Antibodies will bind to the reagent erythrocytes in the incubation period. After removing unbound antibodies by washing the erythrocytes, an anti-IgG AHG reagent is added. And IgG-coated erythrocytes would agglutinate. The IAT for antibodies circulating in the patient's plasma is performed in the following situations:

- Detection of incomplete (nonagglutinating) antibodies to potential donor RBCs (compatibility testing) or screening cells (antibody screen) in serum.
- Determination of RBC phenotype using known antisera (e. g. weak D, any other antigen testing that requires IAT).
- Titration of incomplete antibodies.

Figure 5 - 1 depicts the two variations of the AHG tests: the DAT and the IAT.

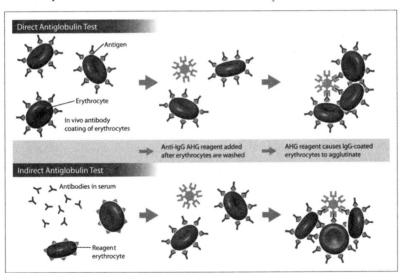

Figure 5 - 1   The direct antiglobulin test (DAT) and indirect antiglobulin test (IAT).
(see Appendix Figure 3)

Zarandona JM, Yazer MH. The role of the Coombs test in evaluating hemolysis in adults [J]. CMAJ. 2006; 174 (3): 305 - 307.

2.1.8   Other techniques

1. Enzymes techniques

Many enzymes can be used in blood group serology, the proteases bromelin, ficin, papain, trypsin, chymotrypsin, neuraminidase, and so on. By cleaving negatively charged sialic acid molecules from polysaccharide chains, the enzymes reduce the red cell surface charge and promote agglutination. Enzyme-treated cells are used in antibody screening and importantly in antibody identification procedures. They are particularly useful for determining specificities within mixtures of antibodies, where one or more are directed against enzyme-sensitive antigens. Enzyme methods are difficult to standardize. Traditionally, enzyme solutions were prepared using a weight-for-volume method. It is necessary to analyze each prepared batch for the activity to ensure standardized tests.

2. Elution techniques

Elution technique is a subsidiary test that may be performed in the elucidation of weak antigens, separation of mixtures of antibodies, detection of causative antibody in HDFN, and investigation of a transfusion reaction or the specificity of an autoantibody in autoimmune hemolytic anaemia (AIHA).

Where an antigen is suspected to be present, but cannot be demonstrated by routine methods, such as Ael and DEL, the cells are incubated with appropriate antibody and the antibody subsequently will be eluted from the cells and identified. An eluate, the product of an elution procedure, can be obtained by using heat, organic solvents such as ether, or by reducing the pH. The eluate can then be subjected to identification procedures.

3. Column-agglutination technology

Column agglutination uses gel or glass beads to trap agglutinated red cells. Red cells are typically allowed to interact with antibodies in chambers at the top of each column. Then the columns or microtubes are centrifuged to force the red cells into the column medium. The column medium, gel or glass beads, then separate agglutinated red cells (which are too large to enter the gel matrix and thus remain at the top of the gel) from nonagglutinated cells that move through the pores in the gel to the bottom of the column. The commercially prepared systems use a card or strip of several microtubes of reactants that allow the performance of several tests simultaneously. The Column agglutination technology can be used to detect the direct agglutination, such as ABO and Rh tests, red cell phenotyping, and for the DAT or IAT.

Besides the techniques mentioned above, some criterions should be noticed. Requests for blood and blood components submitted in electronic, or written format must contain sufficient information for accurate recipient identification (ID). When a pretransfusion specimen is delivered to the laboratory, the laboratory staff must confirm that the information on the specimen label and the pretransfusion testing request are identical. If there is any doubt about the identity of the patient or the labeling of the specimen, a new specimen must be obtained. The strategy prevents the transfusion of incompatible donor red cells that might result in an immune-mediated hemolytic transfusion reaction.

2. 2   Transfusion reactions

Although the overall safety rate of blood transfusion is high, adverse events do still occur. An unfavorable reaction occurs in as many as 1% of transfusions in general. A transfusion reaction can lead to severe discomfort for the patient and an extra cost burden to the health-care system. Although they are rare, reactions can be fatal, with transfusion of about one in 200 000 – 420 000 units associated with death.

2. 2. 1   Defined adverse reactions

- Transfusion-associated circulatory overload (TACO).
- Transfusion-related acute lung injury (TRALI).
- Transfusion-associated dyspnea (TAD).
- Allergic reaction.
- Transfusion-associated hypotension.
- Febrile non-hemolytic transfusion reaction (FNHTR).
- Acute hemolytic transfusion reaction (AHTR).
- Delayed hemolytic transfusion reaction (DHTR).
- Delayed serologic transfusion reaction (DSTR).
- Transfusion-associated graft vs. host disease (TA-GVHD).
- Post-transfusion purpura (PTP).
- Transfusion-transmitted infection (TTI).

The general management for all adverse reaction types is to stop the transfusion, report the transfusion laboratory and keep the intravenous line open with normal isotonic saline; start supportive care to address the patient's cardiac, respiratory, and renal functions as necessary; and provide symptomatic therapy. When the laboratory receives notice of a possible transfusion reaction, several steps are performed by technologists:

- Check the patient sample, component bag, label, and paperwork.
- Repeat ABO testing on the donor and the patient sample, pre-and post-transfusion.
- Direct antiglobulin test (DAT) on a post-transfusion sample.
- Visual check of pre-and post-transfusion samples to look for evidence of hemolysis.
- Report all the findings to the blood bank supervisor or medical director.

2. 2. 2   Febrile non-hemolytic transfusion reaction

Febrile non-hemolytic transfusion reaction (FNHTR) is common, occurring in about 1% of transfusion episodes (1% – 3% per unit transfused). FNHTR is caused by pro-inflammatory cytokines or recipient antibodies encountering donor antigen in the blood product. Reactions clinically present as a temperature rise of 1°C or higher, and can be accompanied by transient hypertension, chills, rigors, and discomfort. In the presence of fever, the transfusion must be stopped immediately and the patient must be assessed closely for signs of infection or hemolysis. Because febrile non-hemolytic reactions are a diagnosis of exclusion, other important transfusion-related aetiologies must be ruled out with post-reaction laboratory evaluation to detect hemolysis (direct antiglobulin test and visual check for grossly haemolysed plasma).

Pre-storage leukocyte reduction can prevent febrile non-hemolytic reactions. Premedication with antipyretics does not decrease the rate of reactions in most patients and should be discouraged. However, the use of antipyretic drugs before transfusion for patients who are persistently febrile due to underlying disease can enable transfusion completion in our experience. The use of platelet additive solutions decreases the rate of reactions from 0.5% to 0.17%.

2.2.3 Acute hemolytic transfusion reaction

Acute hemolytic transfusion reaction (AHTR) can be either immune or non-immune. Immune-mediated acute hemolytic transfusion reactions result from infusion of red blood cells that are incompatible with the patient's anti-A, anti-B, or other red blood cell antibodies. Immune acute hemolytic transfusion reaction is usually caused by failure of patient identification at specimen collection or transfusion, and less commonly by infusion of incompatible plasma, usually from an apheresis platelet transfusion. In either setting, the antigen-antibody interaction can lead to intravascular or extravascular hemolysis, presenting with sudden onset of fever or chills [the most common (80%), and often the only symptom], pain (from kidney capsular distension), hypotension, and dyspnoea. Other signs can include gross hemoglobinuria or hemoglobinaemia, disseminated intravascular coagulation (DIC), acute renal failure, shock, and death. Since fever and chills might be the only early signs, it is important to monitor patients during transfusions and stop the transfusion immediately if there is any change in vital signs or the appearance of unexpected symptoms.

Preventive action programs should target clerical and human errors including patient, sample, and blood unit and reduce the number of such errors.

2.2.4 Allergic reaction

Allergic reaction occurs during or within 4 h of transfusion with a blood component and is most frequently associated with platelet transfusions (302 per 100 000 platelet units). In rare cases, the symptoms may take several hours to develop and cannot be related to blood transfusion. Symptoms are caused by mediators such as histamine, released on activation of mast cells and basophils. Most allergic reactions are mild, with rash, pruritus, urticaria (hives), and localized angio-oedema. When a patient develops mild symptoms, the transfusion should be paused so that an antihistamine, typically 25 to 50 mg diphenhydramine, may be administered. Once the symptoms have evanished, the transfusion can be resumed. The most severe reactions, such as bronchospasm, respiratory distress, and hypotension may also occur. Once a severe reaction or developing anaphylaxis is identified, the transfusion must be stopped and action should be promptly initiated to maintain oxygenation and stabilize hypotension. For patients whose reactions are severe, unrelenting, and unresponsive to premedication, washing red cells or platelets may be considered.

2.2.5   Other transfusion-associated adverse reactions

1. Delayed hemolytic transfusion reaction

Delayed hemolytic transfusion reaction (DHTR) is one kind of delayed transfusion reactions. As with acute transfusion reactions, the consequences of delayed transfusion reactions may be severe but is often treatable. After pregnancy, transfusion, or transplantation, a patient may make an antibody to a red cell antigen. Once the patient subsequently receives a unit of blood expressing the corresponding red cell antigen, red cell antibodies may cause a delayed transfusion reaction. For the hemolysis is primarily extravascular, brisk hemolysis, hemoglobinuria, acute renal failure, and DIC are rare. Unexplained anemia, does not experiences an increase in hemoglobin concentrations following transfusion, jaundice and leukocytosis may develop in these patients.

Approximately 1% to 1.6% of RBC transfusions are associated with antibody formation. Recently transfused or pregnant patients must have samples drawn for compatibility testing within 3 days of the scheduled transfusion to ensure identification of any potential new alloantibodies. To the multiply transfused patients and the patients with sickle cell disease who are easier to develop a complication known as "sickle cell HTR", the transfusion department should have programs to provide at least partially phenotypically matched blood.

The treatment of DHTR consists of monitoring the patient and providing appropriate supportive care. The most frequent therapy is the correction of the anemia by transfusing antigen-negative RBCs as needed.

2. Transfusion-related acute lung injury

Transfusion-related acute lung injury (TRALI) is characterized by the development of non-cardiogenic pulmonary edema after transfusion. Although understanding of the pathogenesis has increased greatly in the past few decades, it remains incompletely understood. Cognate anti-HLA or anti-human neutrophil antigen (anti-HNA) antibodies alone are enough to cause TRALI, but most cases are postulated to occur through a two-event model. The first event is a clinical disorder that causes activation of the pulmonary endothelium, leading to the sequestration and priming of neutrophils in the lung. Clinical risk factors that might function in the first event include high interleukin 8 concentrations, liver surgery, chronic alcohol abuse, shock, high peak airway pressure during mechanical ventilation, current smoking, and positive fluid balance. The second event results from the blood product transfusion, which activates the primed neutrophils causing endothelial damage and subsequent acute lung injury. This can result from either passive transfer of antibodies (immune-mediated) or pro-inflammatory mediators (non-immune mediated) in the transfused component. Since neutrophil sequestration and activation are involved in the development of TRALI, recipient factors including neutrophil number and function also probably play an important role.

The published incidence was varied with the studied patient population and different calculations sources, such as data from National Hemovigilance and Electronic Health Record (EHR) of pulmonary transfusion reactions. It is estimated that the incidence ranges from 0.1% to 8%.

According to AABB standards, blood products from male donors, never-pregnant female donors, or females who have been tested since their last pregnancy and found to be negative for HLA antibodies, can reduce the risk of TRALI.

3. Transfusion-related sepsis

Septic transfusion reactions are usually present during or within 4 h of transfusion. Fever, rigors, hypotension, and other signs associated with systemic inflammatory response syndrome are the most common presentations. In severe cases, the patient may develop shock with accompanying renal failure and DIC. Because of storing at room temperature, platelet units have the highest bacterial contamination rate (one in 3000 – 5000 units); but many do not cause infection because they are removed from the inventory due to positive surveillance, or transfused before bacterial growth has reached a clinically significant level.

Definitive diagnosis of transfusion-transmitted bacterial infection requires isolation of the same organism from the blood product and patient, but can be presumed in a culture-negative patient with clinical sepsis if bacteria are isolated from the transfused unit.

Once transfusion-related sepsis is suspected, the transfusion must be stopped immediately and supportive care of the patient should be initiated. At the same time, both the patient and the remainder of the component should be cultured.

4. Transfusion-associated graft vs. host disease

Transfusion-associated graft vs. host disease (TA-GVHD) is a rare complication of blood transfusion. The clinical manifestations typically begin 8 to 10 days after transfusion, although symptoms can occur as early as 3 days and as late as 30 days. Signs and symptoms include fever, maculopapular rash, enterocolitis with watery diarrhea, liver injury, and pancytopenia. Mortality in TA-GVHD has been estimated to be between 90% and 100%.

There are three possible preconditions involved in the development of TA-GVHD. First, there must be differences in the HLA antigens expressed between the donor and the recipient. Second, immunocompetent cells must be present in the graft. Finally, the host must be incapable of rejecting the immunocompetent cells. The diagnosis of TA-GVHD is based on a combination of characteristic clinical findings, tissue biopsy and molecular techniques. Skin biopsy of these patients can reveal a superficial perivascular lymphocytic infiltrate, necrotic keratinocytes, compact orthokeratosis, and bullae formation. Molecular techniques, such as HLA typing, cytogenetics, and chimerism assessment, specifically donor lymphocytes in recipient tissue, can be used to confirm the diagnosis.

For the disorder is almost uniformly fatal, irradiation of cellular blood components is the only reliable way to prevent it. AABB standards recommend the application of irradiation of cellular blood components when (1) the patient is identified as being at risk of TA-GVHD, (2) the donor is a blood relative of the recipient, and (3) the donor is selected for HLA compatibility by typing or crossmatching.

3   *Discussion*

This case might be one of the transfusion reaction cases in the early time of human beings. Can you recognize the kind of transfusion-associated adverse reaction?

In 1667, Jean Denis, a brilliant young professor of philosophy and mathematics at Montpellier and physician to Louis XIV of France, carried out what is believed to be the first transfusion of animal (lamb's) blood to a human. Antoine Mauroy, an active 34-year-old man who spent some of his time carousing in Paris, was one of his patients. It was thought that blood from a gentle calf might dampen Mauroy's spirits. On December 19, 1667, he received 5 or 6 ounces of blood from the femoral artery of a calf with no untoward effects. Several days later, the procedure was repeated. During the second transfusion, Mauroy experienced pain in the arm receiving the blood, vomiting, increased pulse, a nose bleed, pressure in the chest, and pain over the kidneys; the next day he passed black urine. Two months later, Mauroy died without further transfusions.

References and resources

[1] TAN S Y, GRAHAM C. Karl Landsteiner (1868 – 1943): originator of ABO blood classification [J]. Singapore Med J, 2013, 54 (5): 243 –244.

[2] TIPPETT P A. Speculative model for the Rh blood groups [J]. Annals of human genetics, 1986; 50 (3): 241 –247.

[3] CHEN Q, LI M, LI M, et al. Molecular basis of weak D and DEL in Han population in Anhui Province, China [J]. Chinese medical journal, 2012, 125 (18): 3251 – 3255.

[4] SANDLER SG, CHEN LN, FLEGEL WA. Serological weak D phenotypes: a review and guidance for interpreting the RhD blood type using the RHD genotype [J]. British journal of haematology, 2017, 179 (1): 10 –19.

[5] COOMBS R R, MOURANT A E, RACE R R. A new test for the detection of weak and incomplete Rh agglutinins [J]. British journal of experimental pathology, 1945, 26: 255 – 266.

[6] COOMBS R R, MOURANT A E, RACE R R. In-vivo isosensitisation of red cells in babies with haemolytic disease [J]. Lancet (London, England), 1946, 1 (6391): 264 – 266.

[7] MORESCHI C. Neue Tatsachen über die Blutkorperchen Agglutinationen [J]. Zentralbl Bakteriol, 1908: 46 – 49.

[8] ZARANDONA J M, YAZER M H. The role of the Coombs test in evaluating hemolysis in adults [J]. CMAJ, 2006; 174 (3): 305 – 307.

[9] DELANEY M, WENDEL S, BERCOVITZ R S, et al. Transfusion reactions: prevention, diagnosis, and treatment [J]. Lancet (London, England), 2016, 388 (10061): 2825 – 2836.

[10] BOLTON-MAGGS P H. Bullet points from SHOT: key messages and recommendations from the Annual SHOT Report 2013 [J]. Transfusion medicine (Oxford, England), 2014; 24 (4): 197 – 203.

[11] SANDERS R P, MADDIRALA S D, GEIGER T L, et al. Premedication with acetaminophen or diphenhydramine for transfusion with leucoreduced blood products in children [J]. British journal of haematology, 2005, 130 (5): 781 – 787.

[12] HEDDLE N M. Pathophysiology of febrile nonhemolytic transfusion reactions [J]. Current opinion in hematology, 1999, 6 (6): 420 – 426.

[13] HEDDLE N M, BLAJCHMAN M A, MEYER R M, et al. A randomized controlled trial comparing the frequency of acute reactions to plasma-removed platelets and prestorage WBC-reduced platelets [J]. Transfusion, 2002, 42 (5): 556 – 566.

[14] COHN C S, STUBBS J, SCHWARTZ J, et al. A comparison of adverse reaction rates for PAS C versus plasma platelet units [J]. Transfusion, 2014, 54 (8): 1927 – 1934.

[15] TINEGATE H, BIRCHALL J, GRAY A, et al. Guideline on the investigation and management of acute transfusion reactions. Prepared by the BCSH Blood Transfusion Task Force [J]. British journal of haematology, 2012, 159 (2): 143 – 153.

[16] TOY P, GAJIC O, BACCHETTI P, et al. Transfusion-related acute lung injury: incidence and risk factors [J]. Blood, 2012; 119 (7): 1757 – 1767.

[17] ROUBINIAN N H, TRIULZI D J. Transfusion-associated circulatory overload and transfusion-related acute lung injury: etiology and prevention [J]. Hematology/ oncology clinics of North America, 2019, 33 (5): 767 – 779.

[18] MURPHY W G, COAKLEY P. Testing platelet components for bacterial contamination [J]. Transfus Apher Sci, 2011, 45 (1): 69 – 74.

[19] KATUS M C, SZCZEPIORKOWSKI Z M, DUMONT L J, et al. Safety of platelet transfusion: past, present and future [J]. Vox sanguinis, 2014, 107 (2): 103 – 113.

[20] KOPOLOVIC I, OSTRO J, TSUBOTA H, et al. A systematic review of transfusion-associated graft-versus-host disease [J]. 2015, 126 (3): 406 –414.

[21] GREENWALT TJ. A short history of transfusion medicine [J]. Transfusion, 1997, 37 (5): 550 – 563.

（王立新）

CHAPTER 6
URINE AND OTHER BODY FLUIDS

1 *Words and phrases*

Albuminuria　蛋白尿

Alkaline poisoning　碱中毒

Anuria　无尿症

Bacterialmeningitis　细菌性脑膜炎

Bilirubin　胆红素

Cast　管型

Cerebrospinal fluid　脑脊液

Crystalline　结晶

Dipstick urinalysis　尿干化学分析

Epithelial cell　上皮细胞

Glomerulus　肾小球

Glomerular filtration rate　肾小球滤过率

Glomerulonephritis　肾小球性肾炎

Glycosuria　糖尿

Hematuria　血尿

Hemoglobinuria　血红蛋白尿

Hypotonic urine　低渗尿

Isotonic urine　等渗尿

Ketone　酮体

Ketonemia　酮血症

Ketonuria　酮尿症

Leukocyte esterase　白细胞酯酶

Microscopic examination　显微镜检查

Myoglobinuria　肌红蛋白尿

Nitrite　亚硝酸盐

Nocturia　夜尿

Oliguria　少尿症

Orthostatic proteinuria　体位性蛋白尿

Osmolality　渗透压

Pericardial fluid　心包积液

Peritoneal fluid　腹腔积液

Pleural fluid　胸腔积液

Polyuria　多尿症

Porphyrinuria　卟啉尿

Proteinuria　蛋白尿

Specific gravity　比重

Synovial　滑液的；分泌滑液的

Trichomonas vaginitis　滴虫性阴道炎

Tuberculousmeningitis　结核性脑膜炎

Urine sediment　尿沉渣

Urobilin　尿胆素

Urobilinogen　尿胆原

2　Readings

2.1　Basic examination of urine

Urine is the product of blood passing through the kidneys through glomerular filtration, tubular reabsorption, and secretion.

In normal adults, approximately 1200 mL of blood is perfused into the kidneys per minute, accounting for about 25% of the cardiac output. Each kidney has about 1 million nephrons, which are perfused with blood through the afferent arterioles, and an ultrafiltrate of the plasma passes through each glomerulus into Bowman's space, forming "primary urine". The filtrate is reabsorbed and secreted through the tubules and collecting ducts, where over 99% of various substances such as water and electrolyte were reabsorbed, resulting in urine concentration. In this way, about 180 L "primary urine" can be reduced to 1 - 2 L urine concentration in 24 hours. Ultimately, this urine formed in the kidneys passes from the collecting ducts into the renal pelvis, ureters, bladder, and urethra to be voided. In normal adults, the urine volume is about 1500 mL per 24 hours. The compositions and characteristics of urine can be affected by the functional state of each system of the human body, and therefore reflect the metabolism of the body.

The basic examination of urine consists of four parts: specimen evaluation, physical examination, chemical screening, and sediment examination.

2.1.1   Specimen evaluation

Before one proceeds with any examination, the urine specimen must be evaluated in terms of its acceptability. Considerations include proper labeling, a proper specimen for the requested examination, proper preservative, visible signs of contamination, and whether any transportation delays may have caused significant deterioration.

Urine samples commonly used in clinical practice include first voided morning urine, random urine, timed collection urine, and special urine samples. First voided morning urine is the urine that is discharged for the first time after getting up in the morning, before breakfast and exercising. It generally has stayed in the bladder for 6-8 hours, so it is the most concentrated and best for routine urinalysis. It can be used to evaluate kidney concentrating function, determine human chorionic gonadotropin (hCG) and examine the visible components of erythrocytes, epithelial cells, casts, crystals and tumor cells. Random urine refers to urine samples discharged at any time without any preparation, which is susceptible to the effects of diet, exercise and drugs. Random urine samples are fresh and easy to obtain and suitable for outpatient and emergency screening. For quantitative measurements, timed (12-or 24-hours) urinary collection is preferred for random specimens.

2.1.2   Physical examination

Physical examination is usually a physical character examination, which is the first step of urine examination, including color, clarity, volume, odor, specific, gravity and osmolality.

1. Color

The yellow color of urine is largely due to the pigment urochrome, excretion of which is generally proportional to the metabolic rate. It is increased during fever, thyrotoxicosis, and starvation. Small quantities of urobilin and uroerythrin also contribute to urine coloration. In normal individuals, both pale and dark yellow urine can be produced, and these differences are rough indicators of hydration and urine concentration. Pale urine, typically of low specific gravity, is excreted following high fluid intake; darker urine is seen when fluids are withheld.

The most common abnormal color is red or red-brown. Hematuria (presence of red blood cells), hemoglobinuria, and myoglobinuria may produce pink, red, or red-brown coloration. All of these conditions are easily detectable on reagent strip testing; however, further evaluation is necessary for absolute differentiation. When the blood content of urine reaches or exceeds 1mL per liter, the urine turns reddish or even bright red, which is called macroscopic hematuria. When the blood in urine is very little and the visual color does not change, the number of red blood cells (RBC) per high power field (HPF) is used to define abnormality (>3 RBCs per HPF is defined as microscopic hematuria).

2. Clarity

Urine is normally clear and transparent. The presence of particulate material in the urine specimen produces turbidity, changes the clarity, and warrants further investigation.

The differential diagnosis for cloudy urine is broad, including several nonpathologic entities, cellular elements, and miscellaneous causes. Turbidity may simply be caused by the precipitation of crystals or nonpathologic salts referred to as amorphous substances. Phosphate, ammonium urate, and carbonate can precipitate in alkaline urine, which can be redissolved when acetic acid is added.

The presence of various cellular elements can cause cloudy urine. Leukocytes may form a white cloud similar to that caused by phosphates, but the cloud remains after acidification. Likewise, bacterial growth may cause a uniform opalescence that is not removed by acidification or by filtration, and it has been suggested that turbidimetric assessment using a double-beam turbidimeter may be useful for urine infection screening. Turbidity may also be caused by RBCs, epithelial cells, spermatozoa, or prostatic fluid. Miscellaneous causes for cloudy urine include mucus from the lower urinary tract or genital tract, blood clots, menstrual discharge, and other particulate material such as pieces of tissue, small calculi, clumps of pus, and fecal material.

3. Urine volume

Urine volume refers to the total amount of urine excreted outside the body within 24 hours. The amount of urine depends mainly on the ability of the glomerulus to produce primary urine and the function of concentrating and diluting renal tubules. It is also affected by factors such as spirit, water intake, activity, age, and drugs. Adults produce about 600 − 2000 mL of urine per day, with night urine generally not over 400 mL. Young children, compared with adults, may excrete about three to four times as much urine per kilogram of body weight.

Polyuria is defined as a 24-hour urine volume exceeding 2500 mL. Physiological polyuria refers to polyuria caused by exogenous or physiological factors such as excessive drinking water, food with high water content, intravenous infusion, mental tension, hysteria, etc. It also can occur because of diuretics, caffeine, dehydrants and other drugs. Pathological polyuria is often caused by the dysfunction of renal tubular reabsorption and concentrating, usually occurs in kidney diseases such as the polyuria phase of acute renal failure, the early phase of chronic renal failure, insipidus, primary aldosteronism, hyperthyroidism, and other renal diseases.

Oliguria is the excretion of less than 500 mL of urine per 24 hours, and anuria is the near-complete suppression of urine formation. Physiological oliguria is more common in people with too much sweating or less drinking. Pathological oliguria occurs in the condition of the decreased rate of glomerular filtration caused by renal parenchymal lesions (acute glomerulonephritis, pyelonephritis, etc.), urinary tract obstruction, decreased blood volume or decreased renal blood flow (large area burns, diarrhea, vomiting, excessive hemorrhage, etc).

4. Odor

Urine normally will have a faint and aromatic odor, which is produced by the volatile acids and esters in the urine. Specimens with extensive bacterial overgrowth can be recognized by an ammoniacal and fetid odor. Additionally, eating onions, garlic, curry, leeks, drinking too much, or taking certain drugs can cause a special smell. Ammonia smell is common in chronic cystitis and chronic urinary retention. Garlic smell is found in organophosphate poisoning. Urine in patients with phenylketonuria smells like murine urine. Lack of odor in urine from patients with acute renal failure suggests acute tubular necrosis rather than prerenal failure.

5. Specific gravity and osmolality

The volume of excreted urine and the concentrations of its solutes are varied by the kidney to maintain the homeostasis of body fluid and electrolytes. Specific gravity and osmolality measurements reflect the relative degree of concentration or dilution of a urine specimen. This in turn aids in evaluating the concentrating and diluting abilities of the kidneys.

Specific gravity (SG) refers to the ratio of urine to the same volume of pure water at 4 ℃, reflecting the concentration of solutes contained in urine. Normal adults with adequate fluid intake will produce urine of specific gravity 1.015 − 1.025 over 24 hours; however, normal kidneys can produce urine with a specific gravity that ranges from 1.003 − 1.040. High specific gravity urine is seen in acute nephritis, heart failure, shock, high fever, dehydration or excessive perspiration, diabetes, etc.; low specific gravity urine is seen in acute renal failure, polyuria, chronic renal failure, renal tubulointerstitial disease, acute tubular necrosis, diabetes insipidus, etc.

Osmolality can reflect the relative discharge rate of solutes or water through the kidney, more accurately reflect the function of concentration and dilution of the kidney, and identify renal and pre-renal oliguria. Isotonic urine or hypotonic urine can be found in chronic interstitial lesions such as chronic glomerulonephritis, polycystic kidney disease, obstructive nephropathy, etc.

2.1.3   Chemical screening

Reagent strips are the primary method used for the chemical examination of urine. The chemical measures parameters most commonly found on reagent strips include the potential of hydrogen (pH), protein, glucose, ketones, erythrocyte, bilirubin, urobilinogen, nitrite, leukocyte esterase, vitamin C, etc. Vitamin C is used to determine whether the results of other measures parameters are interfered with by vitamin C.

1. Urine pH

In healthy individuals, random urine pH may vary from 4. 6 − 8 on a normal diet. The principle is the acid-base indicator method. Indicators methyl red and bromothymol blue give a range of orange, green, and blue colors as the pH rises, permitting estimation of pH values within half a unit within the range of 5 − 9.

Urine pH is one of the most important indicators, reflecting the ability of the kidney to regulate the balance of acid-base in the body. Normal fresh urine is often weakly acidic. Alkaline poisoning such as respiratory alkalosis, renal tubular acidosis, and urinary tract infections such as cystitis or pyelonephritis raise the urine pH. In contrast, acidosis, fever, chronic glomerulonephritis, metabolic diseases such as diabetes or gout decrease the urine pH.

2. Protein in urine

Detection of an abnormal amount of protein in urine is an important indicator of renal disease because protein has a very low maximal tubular rate of reabsorption. Normally, up to 150 mg of protein is excreted in the urine daily, with the average urine protein concentration varying from 2 − 10 mg/dL, depending on urine volume. When the urine protein concentration is more than 100 mg/L or 150 mg/24h, the qualitative test of urine protein is positive, naming proteinuria. Proteinuria is composed of albumin in most cases. Detection of urine protein is helpful in early clinical diagnosis and treatment of kidney diseases.

Generally, physiological proteinuria does not have organic pathological changes, often presents as functional proteinuria or orthostatic proteinuria. Functional proteinuria includes mild glomerular proteinuria or mixed proteinuria without renal disease, seen in strenuous exercise, fever, exposure to extreme cold, emotional distress, congestive heart failure, dehydration, etc. The urine protein concentration is usually less than 1 g/24h. Such proteinuria generally has a short duration and will improve with time and appropriate treatment. Orthostatic proteinuria occurs in 3% − 5% of apparently healthy young adults, whose proteinuria only appears when in an upright posture and spinal lordosis, but not lying posture. In this condition, proteinuria is found during the day but not at night when a recumbent position is assumed. For suspected orthostatic proteinuria, two urine specimens should be retained, the first is the morning urine, the second is urine after a few hours of standing. Orthostatic proteinuria can be diagnosed if the urine protein is negative in the first specimen and positive in the second specimen, and the patient should be re-evaluated every 6 months of follow-up.

Overflow proteinuria is due to the overflow of excess levels of a protein in the circulation, which is commonly seen in multiple myeloma immunoglobulin light chain, i. e. Bence-Jones proteinuria, acute phase reaction protein in sepsis, free hemoglobin in hemolysis, and myoglobin in muscle injury. These proteins are not initially associated with glomerular or tubular diseases but may become primary causes of renal damage.

Renal proteinuria can be divided into glomerular proteinuria, tubular proteinuria and mixed proteinuria. Glomerular proteinuria refers to the glomerular damage caused by glomerular disease or other disorders. This type of renal proteinuria is most common and can progress to nephrotic syndrome, with a daily urinary protein of more than 3. 5 g. Tubular proteinuria occurs when tubular reabsorption is altered or impaired, which is associated with the loss of a small amount of urinary protein that would otherwise be largely reabsorbed. Most of these proteins are of low molecular weight, e. g. , α_1-microglobulin, β-globulins such as β_2-microglobulin, light chain immunoglobulins, and lysozyme. The urine reagent strips mainly detect urine albumin, while the ability to detect urine non-albumin is limited, tubular proteinuria may be missed by the reagent strip test because of the absence or very low amounts of albumin. When tubular proteinuria is suspected, the quantitative detection of total urine protein should be performed. Mixed proteinuria refers to the proteinuria produced by simultaneous or successive damage to the glomeruli, and tubules.

Postrenal proteinuria is common in the urinary and reproductive system of inflammation, stones, tuberculosis, and tumors.

3. Glucose in urine

The presence of detectable amounts of glucose in the urine is termed glycosuria. This condition occurs whenever the glucose level in the blood surpasses the renal tubule capacity for reabsorption. Glucose may appear in the urine at different blood glucose levels, and there is not always concomitant hyperglycemia. Glomerular blood flow, tubular reabsorption rate, and urine flow will also influence its appearance. The main factors that contribute to urine glucose include prerenal factors (hyperglycemia) and renal factors (renal tubular reabsorption disorders while blood glucose is normal). Diabetes mellitus is the most common disease that causes hyperglycemia and glycosuria. Urine glucose monitoring plays an important role in the screening, diagnosis, and treatment of diabetes mellitus.

4. Ketones in urine

Ketone is the intermediate product of fat oxidation metabolism. The composition of ketones in the blood and urine is 78% β-hydroxybutyric acid, 20% acetoacetic acid, and 2% acetone. Ketonemia may occur when the rate of ketones production exceeds the tissue utilization rate in the case of glucose metabolism disorders and increased lipolysis. Once the concentration of plasma ketone exceeds the renal threshold (700 mg/L), the urine ketones tests should be positive and ketonuria is formed.

5. Blood, hemoglobin, and myoglobin in urine

The presence of an abnormal number of blood cells in urine is known as hematuria, whereas the term hemoglobinuria refers to the presence of free hemoglobin in urine. Hematuria is relatively common, hemoglobinuria uncommon, and myoglobinuria rare. The presence of free hemoglobin in urine is one of the evidence of intravascular hemolysis, so the urine occult blood test detected by reagent strips is helpful for the diagnosis of intravascular hemolytic diseases.

6. Bilirubin in urine

Bilirubin is a breakdown product of hemoglobin that is formed in the reticuloendothelial cells of the spleen, liver, and bone marrow. Conjugated bilirubin (direct bilirubin) is water-soluble which can pass through the glomerulus of the kidney into the urine. When the concentration of conjugated bilirubin in the blood exceeds the renal threshold, the urinary bilirubin qualitative test should be positive.

Urine bilirubin detection is mainly used for the differential diagnosis of jaundice. Urinary bilirubinis is positive in cholestatic jaundice and hepatocellular jaundice, and is negative in hemolytic jaundice.

7. Urobilinogen in urine

The concentration of urobilinogen in urine is less than 10 mg/L in normal adults. Detection of urinary urobilinogen is helpful for differential diagnosis of different types of jaundice.

Persistent absence of urinary urobilinogen occurs with complete obstruction of the outflow of bile into the intestine, accompanied by pale stools. In contrast, an excess of urobilinogen in the urine together with absent bilirubin is typically associated with hemolysis.

8. Nitrite

Nitrite in urine comes mainly from the reduction reaction of pathogenic microorganisms and the oxidation of nitric oxide (NO) in the body. The urine nitrite test is positive when significant numbers of bacteria is present.

9. Leukocyte esterase

Under normal conditions, only a small amount of white blood cells are contained in the urine, and the qualitative test of leukocyte esterase is negative. However, when the urine contains a large number of neutrophils in the case of infection of the urinary system, the qualitative test of leukocyte esterase is positive.

2.1.4 Sediment examination

The urine-formed elements, also known as urine sediment, are substances that come from the urinary tract, appearing in visible form. The type and/or shape of the urine formed elements varies in different diseases, and even varies in different courses of the same disease. In the routine laboratory, examination of the urine sediment is the best reserved and most useful urine examination when dipstick results are abnormal.

At present, microscopic examination is still regarded as the "gold standard" for morphologic examination of urine sediment. In the microscopic examination, the classification and/or identification of cells, casts, crystals, and other components in urine is an important basis for the localization diagnosis, differential diagnosis, and prognosis evaluation of urinary system diseases.

Importantly, to perform a microscopic evaluation of urine with competence, one must be knowledgeable of numerous morphologic entities (e. g. , organisms, hematopoietic and epithelial cells, crystals, casts). The microscopists can discern subtle alterations in urinary cell morphology, accurately identify cellular and noncellular casts (Figure 9 - 1), and recognize various endogenous and drug-related crystals (Figure 9 - 2). These observations facilitate quick diagnosis of the kidney-related disease processes. As a result, urine sediment examination has been considered as the "liquid biopsy" that provides a window into the kidney. Also, microscopists must be aware of the clinical relevance of urine findings, as well as the common chemical abnormalities associated with microscopic interpretations. Discrepancies should be investigated before a report is issued. The quality of the manual microscopic analysis of urine is dependent on the expertise and experience of the examiner.

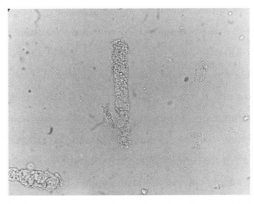

Figure 9 - 1   Protein casts (×400). (see Appendix Figure 4)

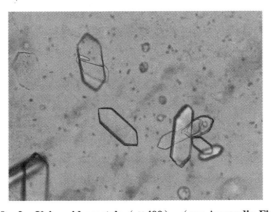

Figure 9 - 2   Uric acid crystals (×400). (see Appendix Figure 5)

In general, randomly collected urine specimens are satisfactory for microscopic examination. It is recommended that examination takes place when the sample is fresh, because cells and casts begin to lyse within 2 hours of collection. Midstream collection is recommended for females to reduce contamination from vaginal elements.

2. 2　Kidney disease and urine testing

The kidneys take part in several regulatory functions. Through glomerular filtration and tubular secretion, numerous waste products, including nitrogenous products of protein catabolism, and both organic and inorganic acids and bases, are eliminated from the body. Fluid, electrolytes (including sodium, potassium, calcium, and magnesium), and acid-base status are regulated in homeostasis. Furthermore, the kidneys provide important hormonal regulation with erythropoietin and renin production, as well as vitamin D activation. Any derangement of these functions by the renal or systemic disease can be reflected as chemically or cytologically altered urine.

Abnormal changes in urine character and composition can occur in the early stage of kidney disease. Structural damage to the kidneys at different locations can lead to different changes in the urine. For example, when the glomerular injury appears, if only the glomerular filtration membrane charge barrier is damaged, it can cause medium molecular proteins such as albumin and transferrin to filter into the urine, which is called selective proteinuria. When the glomerular filtration membrane aperture barrier is damaged, large, medium, and small molecular proteins can filter into the urine, which is called non-selective proteinuria. When the glomerular basement membrane is ruptured, red blood cells can also pass through the glomerular filtration membrane to form glomerular hematuria, where red blood cells and red blood cell casts may appear in the urine. If the renal tubule is injured, when the injury occurs in the proximal tubule, it mainly affects the reabsorption dysfunction, causing small molecule proteinuria, glycosuria, amino acid urine, and increased urine bicarbonate; when the injury occurs in the medullary loops and distal tubules, it leads to the dysfunction of renal concentration and dilution, resulting in hypotonic urine, polyuria and nocturia, and acid-base disbalance.

2. 2. 1　Acute glomerulonephritis

Acute glomerulonephritis is more common in children, the onset of the disease is more urgent. The main clinical features include hematuria, proteinuria, hypertension, edema, oliguria, and azotemia. Hematuria is often the earliest clinical symptom of acute glomerulonephritis. In the urine of patients with acute glomerulonephritis, deformable erythrocytes can be found by urine erythrocyte morphology examination, presenting as anisocytosis, acanthocyte, ring erythrocytes, etc.

Almost all the patients with acute glomerulonephritis are positive for qualitative urine protein testing, but the degree is generally not serious. The urine protein quantity is mostly 0.5 - 3.0g per day, and less than 20% of the patients have urine protein quantity greater than 3.5g per day, most of which are non-selective proteinuria.

Creatinine is the metabolite of phosphocreatine in human muscles, which is the only source of creatinine in the human body. In the case of a strict diet, the body's endogenous creatinine production is equal to urine output every day, and relatively constant. Creatinine is primarily filtered through the glomeruli and is not reabsorbed by the tubules. The endogenous creatinine clearance (Ccr) refers to the amount of plasma that can be processed when the kidney removes all creatinine from certain plasma and excretes it into urine every minute. Endogenous creatinine clearance is an early indicator of renal damage, and it is one of the best renal function tests commonly used in clinical practice because of its simple operation, less interference, and higher sensitivity. In acute glomerulonephritis, the endogenous creatinine clearance can be less than 80% of the reference range while serum creatinine and urea are in the reference range.

2.2.2   Rapidly progressive glomerulonephritis

Rapidly progressive glomerulonephritis is a group of glomerular diseases, which is characterized by acute nephritis syndrome, rapid deterioration of renal function, early onset of oliguria and other acute renal failure. The pathologic feature of rapidly progressive glomerulonephritis is cresentic glomerulonephritis.

Rapidly progressive glomerulonephritis may present with a sharp deterioration in renal function within a day to weeks, also with oliguria and anuria. Urine is collected for 24 hours and the urine volume is measured, oliguria (Urine Volume≤400 mL per day) or anuria (Urine Volume ≤ 100 mL per day) can occur in the early stages of rapidly progressive glomerulonephritis. Due to the frequent secondary renal tubulointerstitial damage, the urinary specific gravity of patients with rapidly progressive glomerulonephritis is less than 1.020.

Similar to acute glomerulonephritis, patients with rapidly progressive glomerulonephritis often have deformed erythrocytes and erythrocyte casts in the urine. However, gross hematuria can be seen in most cases of rapidly progressive glomerulonephritis, with a large number of red blood cells visible under the microscope. This is more severe than acute glomerulonephritis and it usually deteriorates continuously, and the number of white blood cells in the urine is often increased too, mostly neutrophils and monocytes.

In patients with rapidly progressive glomerulonephritis, serum creatinine and urea are elevated, and the endogenous creatinine clearance may decrease significantly without any improvement.

2.2.3   Chronic glomerulonephritis

Chronic nephritis syndrome refers to a group of glomerular diseases with proteinuria, hematuria, hypertension, and edema as the basic clinical manifestations, which can have different degrees of renal hypofunction and eventually develop into chronic renal failure.

Chronic glomerulonephritis is the main cause of chronic nephritis syndrome, and its pathological types include mesangial proliferative glomerulonephritis, membranoproliferative glomerulonephritis, membranous nephropathy, focal stage glomerulonephritis, etc. However, as the disease progresses, patients with chronic glomerulonephritis gradually develop into glomerulosclerosis, renal tubular atrophy, and renal interstitial fibrosis, which lead to chronic and irreversible renal impairment. Chronic glomerulonephritis patients, often with a long asymptomatic period, may only present as microalbuminuria in the early stage, and then gradually develop to mild /moderate proteinuria and renal abnormalities. The basic clinical manifestations of patients with chronic glomerulonephritis are hematuria, proteinuria, and edema, and gradually develop to chronic renal failure.

Proteinuria is the most important clinical manifestation of chronic glomerulonephritis. Generally, the level of urinary protein in patients with chronic glomerulonephritis is in the range of 1 - 3g per day, and some patients may present with macroproteinuria (greater than 3.5g per day). The higher the level of urinary protein, the longer the duration of proteinuria, the worse the prognosis. But when the patients progress to kidney failure, the urine protein decreases.

In the early stage of chronic renal damage, such as chronic glomerulonephritis, when the amount of damaged glomeruli is small and the degree of damage is mild, the level of urinary albumin can exceed the upper limit of the reference (20 mg/L), However, it still cannot reach the lowest detection limit of conventional methods (200 mg/L), which is called microalbuminuria. Urinary microalbumin is a sensitive and reliable indicator for the early diagnosis of chronic glomerulonephritis.

β_2-microglobulin and α_1-microglobulin are low molecular proteins, which are sensitive and specific indicators of tubular lesions. In the early stages of chronic glomerulonephritis, urine levels of both proteins can be significantly elevated, suggesting tubular damages.

2.3 Nephrotic syndrome

Nephrotic syndrome is a group of diseases characterized by massive proteinuria (> 3.5g per day), hypoproteinemia (< 30g/L), edema, and hyperlipidemia.

Massive proteinuria is the primary characteristic of nephrotic syndrome, and it can lead to increased urine specific gravity. Minimal change nephropathy is mainly characterized by selective proteinuria, in which urine proteinuria electrophoresis presents medium molecular weight proteinuria, such as albumin and transferrin. The urine protein of other primary nephropathy patients is usually non-selective. In addition to medium molecular weight protein, there are IgG, complement C3 and other macromolecular proteins. When lesions involve proximal renal tubules, the levels of small molecular weight proteins such as β_2 - microglobulin in the urine may also exceed the reference range.

The incidence and severity of hematuria in patients with the nephrotic syndrome also vary according to the types of pathology. Minimal change nephropathy generally has no gross hematuria, and the incidence of microscopic hematuria is about 15% − 20%. The incidence of hematuria in mesangial proliferative glomerulonephritis is higher, with gross hematuria up to 30% − 60% and microscopic hematuria up to 70% − 100%. Gross hematuria is seen in about 20% of mesangial capillary glomerulonephritis, but microscopic hematuria is present in almost 100%. There are various types of casts in the urine of patients with nephrotic syndrome.

3   *Discussion*

A 10-year-old boy visited the doctor because of hematuria and facial edema for 2 days. The doctor's initial diagnosis of the patient was acute glomerulonephritis. What abnormalities should be presented in the basic examination of urine to support this diagnosis?

Resources and references

[1] 彭明婷. 临床血液与体液检验 [M]. 北京：人民卫生出版社，2017.

[2] MCPHERSON R A , PINCUS M R. Henry's clinical diagnosis and management by laboratory methods [M]. 22nd ed. Philadelphia：Elsevier, 2011.

（郑　沁）

CHAPTER 7

ACUTE MYELOID LEUKEMIA

1 *Words and phrases*

Hematopoietic 造血的

Myeloid 髓系的

Lymphoid 淋巴的

Histiocytic 组织细胞的

Neoplasm 肿瘤

Provisional 暂定的，临时的

Homogeneous 同质的，同种类的

Heterogeneous 异质的，各种各样的

Acute myeloid leukemia（AML） 急性髓性白血病

Acute lymphoblastic leukemia（ALL） 急性淋巴细胞白血病

Acute leukemia of ambiguous lineage（ALAL） 不明谱系的急性白血病

Blastic plasmacytoid dendritic cell neoplasm（BPDCN）
母细胞性浆细胞样树突状细胞肿瘤

Myeloproliferative neoplasm（MPN） 骨髓增殖性肿瘤

Myelodysplastic syndrome（MDS） 骨髓增生异常综合征

Morphology 形态学

Cytogenetic 细胞遗传学的

Immunophenotype 免疫表型

Multiparameter flow cytometry 多参数流式细胞分析

Immunohistochemistry 免疫组织化学

FMS-related tyrosine kinase 3（FLT3） FMS 相关的酪氨酸激酶 3

Internal tandem duplication（ITD） 近膜结构域内部串联重复

Karyotype 核型

Next-generation sequencing（NGS） 下一代测序

Allogeneic hematopoietic stem cell transplantation（allo-HSCT）

异体造血干细胞移植

De novo 原发的

Progeny 后代

Exertional 劳力的

Pallor 皮肤苍白

Thrombocytopenia 血小板减少症

Hemorrhage 出血

Neutropenia 中性粒细胞减少症

Monocytopenia 单核细胞减少症

Blast 原始细胞

Acute megakaryoblastic leukemia 急性巨核细胞白血病

Acute myelomonocytic leukemia 急性粒单核细胞白血病

Acute promyelocytic leukemia 急性早幼粒细胞白血病

Monoblastic 原始单核细胞的

Myelofibrosis 骨髓纤维化

Myeloid sarcoma 粒细胞肉瘤

All-trans-retinoic acid 全反式视黄酸

Autologous stem cell infusion 自体干细胞输注

Measurable residual disease（MRD） 微小残留疾病

Risk stratification 危险度分层

Whole exome sequencing 全外显子测序

Whole genome sequencing 全基因组测序

Somatic coding mutation 体细胞编码突变

Cellular immunotherapy 细胞免疫疗法

Graft-versus-host disease（GVHD） 移植物对抗宿主疾病

Immunosuppression 免疫抑制

Adoptive cellular therapy（ACT） 输入细胞疗法

Chimeric antigen receptor（CAR） 嵌合抗原受体

Complete remission（CR） 完全缓解

2　Readings

2. 1　Diagnosis in tumors of the hematopoietic and lymphoid tissues：the art of distinction

2. 1. 1　World Health Organization recommendations

The World Health Organization（WHO）classification classifies neoplasms primarily according to lineage: myeloid, lymphoid, or histiocytic/dendritic, and a normal counterpart is postulated for each neoplasm. Most of the diseases described in the WHO classification are considered to be distinct entities; however, some are not as clearly defined and listed as provisional entities. In addition, borderline categories have been created for cases that do not clearly fit into a single category, so that well-defined categories can be kept homogeneous and borderline cases can be studied further. Although the goal is to define the lineage of each neoplasm, lineage plasticity can occur in precursor or immature neoplasms, and has also been identified in some mature hematolymphoid neoplasms. In addition, genetic abnormalities, such as rearrangements in FGFR1, PDGFRA, and PDGFRB, or PCM1-JAK2 fusion, can give rise to neoplasms of either myeloid or lymphoid lineage associated with eosinophilia; these disorders are recognized as a separate group. Precursor neoplasms [i.e. acute myeloid leukemias (AML), lymphoblastic leukemias / lymphomas (ALL/LBL), acute leukemias of ambiguous lineage (ALAL), and blastic plasmacytoid dendritic cell neoplasm (BPDCN)] are discussed separately from more mature neoplasms [i.e. myeloproliferative neoplasms (MPN), mastocytosis, myelodysplastic syndromes (MDS), mature B-cell and T/NK-cell neoplasms, Hodgkin lymphomas (HL), histiocytic / dendritic cell neoplasms]. The mature myeloid neoplasms are classified by their biological features (i.e. MPN with effective hematopoiesis vs. MPN with ineffective hematopoiesis), as well as by their genetic features. Within the category of mature lymphoid neoplasms, the diseases are generally listed according to their clinical presentation (i.e. disseminated, often leukemic, extranodal, indolent, or aggressive), and to some extent according to the stage of differentiation when this can be postulated.

2.1.2 Laboratory diagnosis: MICM classification

Nowadays, morphology (M), immunology (I), cytogenetic (C) and molecular biology (M) classification is of significance in the diagnosis of many tumors of the hematopoietic and lymphoid tissues. Morphology is always important. The availability of immunophenotype and genetic features help much more in establishing consensus definitions than it was when only subjective morphological criteria were available. Immunophenotyping can be utilized both to determine lineage in malignant processes and to distinguish between benign and malignant processes. Immunophenotypic analysis by either multiparameter flow cytometry or immunohistochemistry using peripheral blood, bone marrow, and lymph node samples is an essential tool in the characterization of neoplasms. Also, a specific genetic abnormality may be the key defining criterion. Some genetic abnormalities are characteristic of a given disease or disease group but not specific, such as MYC, CCND1, and BCL2 rearrangements and JAK2 mutations; others are prognostic factors for several diseases, such as TP53 mutations and FLT3 internal tandem duplication (FLT3-ITD). Moreover, the frequent use of immunophenotypic features and genetic abnormalities to define entities has also enabled the identification of antigens, genes, and pathways that can be targeted for therapy. The best examples include the success of the anti-CD20 monoclonal antibody rituximab for the treatment of B-cell neoplasms and the success of the tyrosine kinase inhibitor imatinib for the treatment of leukemias associated with rearrangements in *ABL1* and other tyrosine kinase genes. Furthermore, a number of disease entities in the WHO classification are defined in part by specific genetic abnormalities, including gene rearrangements due to chromosomal translocations, deletions, and specific gene mutations; therefore, a complete cytogenetic analysis of the bone marrow by either conventional karyotyping or by the newly emerging array-based and next-generation sequencing (NGS) technologies should be performed at the time of initial evaluation to establish the cytogenetic profile and at regular intervals thereafter to detect evidence of genetic evolution. Finally, the diagnosis of some diseases requires knowledge of clinical features such as patient age, nodal versus extranodal presentation, specific anatomical site, and history of cytotoxic and other therapies.

2.2 Acute myeloid leukemia

2.2.1 Definition

Acute myeloid leukemia (AML) is a malignant disorder of hematopoietic tissues characterized by clonal expansion and differentiation of leukemic myeloid blast cells, principally in the marrow, and impaired production of normal blood cells. AML is the most common form of acute leukemias in adults with the shortest survival (5-year survival 24%). Curative therapies, including intensive chemotherapy and allogeneic hematopoietic stem cell transplantation (allo-HSCT), are generally applicable to a minority of patients who are younger and fit, while older individuals tend to exhibit poor prognosis and survival. Differences in patient outcomes are influenced by disease characteristics, access to care including active therapies and supportive care, as well as other factors.

2.2.2 Etiology

AML is the result of sequential somatic mutations in a primitive multipotential hematopoietic cell. The pathophysiology of AML is rooted in the genetic perturbation of hematopoietic progenitor cells, which ultimately favors the clonal and malignant expansion of immature myeloblasts. Such are deemed leukemia-initiating cells or leukemic stem cells and prompt the ineffective hematopoiesis and other pathology with which the disease manifests. In comparison to de novo AML, secondary AML is an inclusive description of AML that arises out of DNA damage induced by prior exposure to chemotherapy or radiotherapy [therapy-related AML (t-AML)], prior non-therapeutic, toxic exposures or prior hematologic malignancy. A small but increasing proportion of cases develop after a patient with lymphoma, a non-hematologic cancer, or an autoimmune disorder exposed to intensive chemotherapy, especially with alkylating agents or topoisomerase Ⅱ inhibitors. Secondary AML comprises 10% −30% of all

AML with the t-AML subset comprising 7% − 15% of all AML.

2. 2. 3   Pathogenesis and laboratory manifestations

The mutant hematopoietic cell acquires the features of a leukemic stem cell capable of self-renewal and desultory differentiation and maturation. It gains a growth and survival advantage in relationship to the normal polyclonal pool of hematopoietic stem cells. As the progeny of this mutant, now leukemic, multipotential cell proliferates continuously, normal hematopoiesis is inhibited, and normal red cell, neutrophil, and platelet blood levels fall. Thus, the leukemic cell infiltration in marrow is accompanied, nearly invariably, by anemia and thrombocytopenia. The resultant anemia leads to weakness, exertional limitations, and pallor; the thrombocytopenia to spontaneous hemorrhage, usually in the skin and mucous membranes; and the neutropenia and monocytopenia to poor wound healing and minor infections. Severe infection usually does not occur at diagnosis, but often does if the disease progresses because of lack of treatment or if chemotherapy intensifies the decrease of blood neutrophil and monocyte levels.

2. 2. 4   Classification

The current categorization of AML is guided by the WHO recommendations (Table 7 − 1).

Table 7 − 1   World Health Organization Classification of AML and Related Precursor Neoplasm.

AML with recurrent genetic abnormalities
AML with t (8; 21) (q22; q22. 1); *RUNX1-RUNX1T1*
AML with inv (16) (p13. 1q22) or t (16; 16) (p13. 1; q22); *CBFB-MYH*11
Acute promyelocytic leukemia with t (15; 17) (q11 − 12); *PML-RARA*
AML with t (9; 11) (p21. 3; q23. 3); *KMT2A-MLLT*3
AML with t (6; 9) (p23; q34. 1); *DEK-NUP*214
AML with inv (3) (q21. 3q26. 2) or t (3; 3) (q21. 3; q26. 2); *GATA2, MECOM*
AML (megakaryoblastic) with t (1; 22) (p13. 3; q13. 1); *RBM15-MKL*1
AML with *BCR-ABL*1
AML with gene mutations
AML with mutated *NPM*1
AML with biallelic mutation of *CEBPA*
AML with mutated *RUNX*1
AML with myelodysplasia-related changes
Therapy-related acute myeloid neoplasms

(To be countinued)

(Continued)

AML, not otherwise specified
AML with minimal differentiation
AML without maturation
AML with maturation
Acute myelomonocytic leukemia
Acute monoblastic and monocytic leukemia
Pure erythroid leukemia
Acute megakaryoblastic leukemia
Acute basophilic leukemia
Acute panmyelosis with myelofibrosis
Myeloid sarcoma
Myeloid proliferations associated with Down syndrome
Transient abnormal myelopoiesis associated with Down syndrome
Myeloid leukemia associated with Down syndrome

2. 2. 5   Diagnostics

The diagnosis of AML is based on identification and measurement of leukemic blast cells in the blood and marrow, which further classifies the cases into distinct biologically groups based on morphology, clinical features, immunophenotype, cytogenetic and molecular abnormalities under the guidance of the WHO recommendations. However, approximately one-third of new AML diagnoses are made without manual bone marrow aspirate blast counts, but rather estimated by bone marrow flow cytometric analysis or immunohistochemistry. Because the leukemic stem cell is capable of imperfect differentiation and maturation, the clone may contain cells with the morphologic or immunophenotypic features of erythroblasts, megakaryocytes, monocytes, eosinophils, or, rarely, basophils or mast cells, in addition to myeloblasts or promyelocytes. When one cell line is sufficiently dominant, the leukemia may be referred to by that lineage: for example, acute erythroid, acute megakaryocytic, acute monocytic leukemia, etc. Certain cytogenetic alterations are more frequent; these abnormalities include t (8; 21), t (15; 17), inversion 16 or t (16; 16), trisomy 8, and deletions of all or part of chromosome 5 or 7. A translocation involving chromosome 17 at the site of the retinoic acid receptor-α (RAR-α) gene is uniquely associated with acute promyelocytic leukemia. Despite of expert panel's recommendation, molecular testing for the presence of even common mutations is not undertaken for 100% of the cases. In summary, the current diagnosis and work-up of AML are not standardized and vary in different practice settings and by different practitioners.

Increasing awareness of these diagnostic inadequacies and disparities is necessary to foster the increased use of recommended testing and thus optimal risk stratification for AML patients.

2.2.6 Treatment

Today, AML is primarily defined according to leukemia-cell karyotype and an increasing number of molecular aberrations. It follows that different types of AML should ideally be treated differently. AML is usually treated with cytarabine and an anthracycline antibiotic, although other drugs may be added or substituted in poor-prognosis, older, refractory, or relapsed patients. The exception to this approach is the treatment of acute promyelocytic leukemia with all-trans-retinoic acid, arsenic trioxide, and sometimes an anthracycline antibiotic. High-dose chemotherapy and either autologous stem cell infusion or allo-HSCT may be used in an effort to treat relapse or patients at high risk to relapse after chemotherapy treatment. After accounting for various confounding factors, complete response with cytotoxic therapy is associated with longer remissions and survival than complete remission with incomplete count recovery. Indeed, since patients in complete remission but with flow cytometric, cytogenetic, or molecular evidence of measurable residual disease have worse outcomes than patients in complete remission without measurable residual disease (MRD), these two groups of patients with AML are now commonly considered to be distinct entities. In summary, biologically-distinct subtypes of AML have variable prognoses, and sociodemographic and healthcare factors influence the care of AML patients and consequently their survival.

2.3 Extended reading

2.3.1 Next-generation sequencing

Next-generation sequencing (NGS) enables reliable detection of patient-specific mutations covering complete genes in molecularly heterogeneous diseases such as AML. According to the 2017 European Leukemia Net (ELN) recommendations, NGS should be incorporated in the routine work-up of preferably bone marrow specimens for accurate risk stratification in AML. A number of commercially available gene panels focusing on genes frequently mutated in myeloid malignancies have been introduced, e. g. the Illumina Trusight Myeloid panel, the Archer Variant Plex Core Myeloid panel, the Human Myeloid Neoplasms QIASeq DNA panel and the AmpliSeq for Illumina Myeloid panel. These panels contain all genes relevant for the 2017 ELN classification and show an enormous overlap in additional mutational hotspots and complete coverage of genes frequently mutated in myeloid diseases. In addition to these commercial panels, gene panels can be easily configured to meet local requirements. Since most of the clinically relevant mutations in myeloid malignancies are known, targeted sequencing is currently the method of primary choice. However, the use of whole exome or whole genome sequencing will allow identification of all somatic coding mutations, including those that are targetable but less frequently present in AML. Moreover, one can prioritize analysis of key AML genes first, such that initial results regarding the clinically most relevant genes can be obtained with a short turnaround and more comprehensive genomic profiling can follow later. Furthermore, whole genome sequencing allows identification of novel biomarkers located outside of protein coding regions, which may be useful not only for proper assessment of the prognosis but also for detection of MRD in AML as they can be used to identify and follow leukemic clones regardless of their role in AML initiation and maintenance.

In fact, MRD detection is of substantial value in predicting relapse and overall survival when applied to AML in complete remission, however, the use of molecular enumeration of MRD has been limited to only specific, molecularly defined subtypes of AML. Recent studies have shown that a variety of more sensitive laboratory methods, including NGS measuring submicroscopic MRD other than morphologic assessment of the percentage of bone marrow myeloblasts, can be utilized as consistent, independent prognostic factors for AML relapse and survival. NGS simultaneously assesses mutations in most AML driver mutations, thus the vast majority of patients will have a trackable mutation at diagnosis that can serve as an applicable MRD marker. Recently, it has been shown that molecular MRD detection by NGS is applicable to virtually every newly diagnosed AML patient because of the frequent prevalence of multiple molecular aberrations among patients with AML. Currently, the major limitations of the NGS-based methodology of detecting MRD are related to the limited sensitivity and specificity of the assays and the inability to discriminate correctly between residual leukemia and clonal hematopoiesis. It is important to recognize that both commercial NGS-based assays and those developed in-house as well as downstream analyses should be thoroughly validated locally before implementation in daily practice.

2.3.2 Cellular immunotherapy

Current chemotherapy-based treatment of AML is associated with significant toxicity and morbidity. Allo-HSCT is the only potentially curative intervention, However, it is also associated with considerable morbidity and mortality due to graft-versus-host disease (GVHD) and complications of immunosuppression. Adoptive cellular therapy (ACT) interventions may provide more profound responses through specific targeting of malignant cells. Different forms of ACTs have been clinically tested for AML, but the progresses were limited by the number of treated patients, treatment-associated toxicities, low clinical responses, or difficulties in identifying suitable targets. Significant improvements in the survival of patients with hematological cancers following allo-HSCT provide evidence for the potency of immune cell-mediated anti-leukemic effects. Studies focusing on immune cell-based cancer therapies have made significant breakthroughs in the last few years. ACT, and chimeric antigen receptor (CAR)-T cell therapy, in particular, have significantly increased the survival of patients with B cell acute lymphoblastic leukemia and aggressive B cell lymphoma. With CAR-T therapy, complete remission (CR) rates of up to 90% have been achieved in refractory or relapsed CD19[+] B cell acute lymphoblastic leukemia (B-ALL), where the expected response rate is approximately 30% with conventional chemotherapy. AML is a clinically heterogeneous disease with numerous genetic mutations and chromosomal abnormalities. The findings of the successes of CD19-CAR-T cells are not directly translatable to AML due to its distinct characteristics. While some cancer types have common tumor-associated antigens that are easier to target, no ubiquitous and targetable common cancer antigens have been identified for a heterogeneous disease like AML. A minority of AML patients have mutations that lead to antigenic fusion proteins and mutant tumor-specific proteins (e. g. AML1-ETO, FLT3, NPM1), which can act as leukemia-specific antigens (LSAs). Many other non-specific antigens but preferentially expressed on leukemic cells are considered as leukemia-associated antigens (LAAs), e. g. Wilms' tumor protein 1 (WT1), which may serve as targetable antigens. The current clinical trials using ACT in an antigen-specific manner to target LSAs, LAAs, or other antigenic targets for treating AML patients include WT-1 Trans-genic Auto-TCR-T cells, WT1-specific CD8[+] Allo-CTLs, CD33 Auto-CAR-T cells, WT1-dendritic cells (DC) and so on. As an alternative approach, cells that recognize AML in an antigen-nonspecific manner, such as natural killer (NK) cells, gamma-delta T cells, cytokine-induced killer (CIK) cells, and double negative T (DNT) cells can be developed as an ACT. Further and more active investigations in diverse approaches of ACTs are needed to take full advantage of the therapeutic potential of ACT against AML.

Due to the highly heterogeneous properties of AML within and among patients, sharing of myeloid lineage markers with HSCs, and existing immune-escape mechanisms, targeting a single antigen to achieve significant clinical benefits across AML populations may be challenging. The use of antigen-nonspecific approaches may be more feasible; however, their relatively low potency needs to be improved in order to achieve better outcomes. Researchers are combining antigen-specific and antigen-nonspecific approaches as a way to optimize cellular immunotherapies, which has shown some promising results. While initial attempts to use CAR technology for cell therapy have focused on T cells, there are growing interests in using innate immune cells as CAR carriers. For example, CD123-CARs with 4-1BB co-stimulatory and CD3 signaling domains have been transduced on NK92 cell lines to avoid T cell-associated toxicities while maximizing the therapeutic benefits of CARs. Therefore, to enhance ACTs for a broader AML patient population, studies to improve upon their respective weaknesses will be needed to minimize on-target off-tumor toxicities for antigen-specific therapies and increase the anti-leukemic potency for antigen-nonspecific therapies. For patients who cannot tolerate the high toxicity of antigen-specific ACTs, antigen-nonspecific ACTs may be more suitable due to their relatively low treatment-associated toxicity, whereas for patients with aggressive disease, therapeutic benefits from the high potency of antigen-specific ACTs may outweigh some degree of their associated toxicities. Further investigation of their efficacy and safety in a clinical setting is needed.

3 *Discussion*

Read the following case description, learn the clinical approach to APL and translate the case note into Chinese.

The patient is a 57-year-old man with pancytopenia in CBC routine test (Hb 51 g/L, PLT 16 × 10^9/L, WBC 0.34 × 10^9/L). He was referred to a hematologist and bone marrow aspiration for further tests was ordered.

Morphology: Bone marrow smear showed a high percentage of myeloid cells of 76.5%, and 74% were promyelocytes with abnormal morphology. The abnormal cells were of medium-size and irregular shape. The nuclei were kidney-shaped or bilobed. The cytoplasm was marked by densely packed or even coalescent large granules, staining light blue. The cytoplasmic granules were large and numerous. Individual cells containing bundles of Auer rods randomly distributed within the cytoplasm were present.

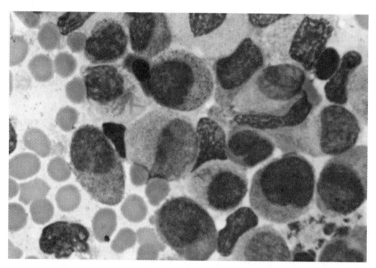

Figure 7 − 1   Bone marrow morphology. (see Appendix Figure 6)

Cytochemistry: The MPO reaction was always strongly positive in all the leukemic promyelocytes, with the reaction product covering the entire cytoplasm and often the nucleus.

Immunophenotyping: For multiparameter flow cytometry based immunophenotyping, the abnormal cells showed expression of CD117, homogeneous bright expression of CD33, and heterogeneous expression of CD13 and strong expression of cytoplasmic MPO (CMPO), absent expression of HLA-DR and CD34.

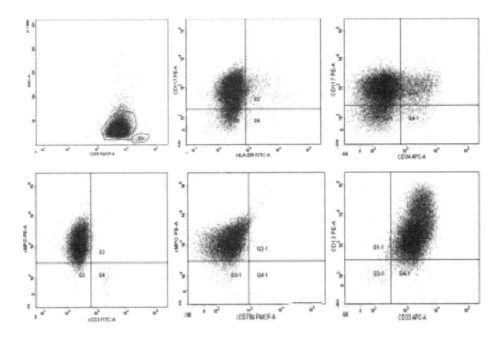

Figure 7 − 2   Multiparameter flow cytometry analysis of bone marrow aspiration.

(**see Appendix Figure 7**)

Cells were stained in tube 1 with FITC-HLA-DR/PE-CD117/APC-CD34/PerCP-CD45, tube 2 with FITC-CD3/PE-MPO/APC-CD45/PerCP-CD79a (for cytosol CD3, MPO and CD79a detection) and tube 3 PE-CD13/APC-CD33/PerCP-CD45

Cytogenetics: A classic t (15; 17) (q24. 1; q21. 2) karyotype on routine cytogenetic study was described with complex variant translocations involving chromosomes 15 and 17.

Molecular Biology: PML-RARα fusion gene product was detected.

Laboratory Diagnosis: The characteristic MICM suggest acute promyelocyte leukemia (APL).

Resources and references

[1] KAUSHANSKY K, LICHTMAN M A, PRCHAL JT. Williams hematology [M] 9th ed. Sykesville: McGraw-Hill Medical, 2015.

[2] SWERDLOW S H, CAMPO E, HARRIS N L, et al. WHO classification of tumours of haematopoietic and lymphoid tissues (revised 4th edition)   [M]. Geneva: WHO Press, 2008.

[3] LEVINE R L, VALK P J M. Next-generation sequencing in the diagnosis and minimal residual disease assessment of acute myeloid leukemia [J]. Haematologica, 2019, 104 (5): 868 − 871.

[4] SHALLIS R M, WANG R, DAVIDOFF A, et al. Epidemiology of acute myeloid leukemia: recent progress and enduring challenges [J]. Blood Reviews, 2019, 36:

70 - 87.

[5] LEE J B, CHEN B, VASIC D, et al. Cellular immunotherapy for acute myeloid leukemia: How specific should it be? [J]. Blood Reviews, 2019, 35: 18 - 31.

[6] ESTEY E. Acute myeloid leukemia—many diseases, many treatments [J]. N Engl J Med, 2016, 375 (21): 2094 - 2095.

(廖红艳)

CHAPTER 8
THERAPEUTIC DRUG MONITORING

1 *Words and phrases*

Acetylator phenotype 乙酰化表型

Administration of the drug 给药

Antagonistic 拮抗的，对抗的

Antiarrhythmic drug 抗心律失常药物

Antibiotic 抗生素

Antiepileptic drug 抗癫痫药物

Antifungal drug 抗真菌药物

Antipsychotic drug 抗精神病药物

Anti-tumor drug 抗肿瘤药物

Area under the concentration-time curve（AUC） 浓度－时间曲线下面积

Bioavailability 生物利用度

Biotransformation 生物转运

Chemiluminescence 化学发光

Chromatography 色谱分析

Cross-reactant 交叉反应物

Dosage 剂量

Dose-response curve 剂量－效应曲线

Drug interaction 药物相互作用

Elimination 消除

Empirically 以经验为主地，经验主义地

Enantiomer 立体异构体

First-pass effect 首过效应

Half-life of the drug 药物半衰期

Heterogeneous 非均相的

Homogeneous 均相的

Immunoassay　免疫分析

Immunosuppressive drug　免疫抑制剂

Liquid chromatography-mass spectrum（LC-MS）　液相色谱－质谱

Limited sampling strategies（LSSs）　有限抽样策略

Maintenance dosage　维持剂量

Mass spectrometry　质谱

Non-linear pharmacokinetics　非线性药代动力学

Optical absorbance　光吸收度

Overdose　超剂量

Patient compliance　患者依从性

Peak concentration　峰浓度

Placebo effect　安慰剂效应

Route of administration　给药途径

Steady state　稳态

Synergistic　协同的，协作的

Therapeutic drug monitoring（TDM）　治疗药物监测

Therapeutic index　治疗指数

Tissue responsiveness　组织应答

Trough concentration　谷浓度

Fluorescence polarization immunoassay（FPIA）　荧光偏振免疫分析

Enzyme-multiplied immunoassay technique（EMIT）　酶放大免疫分析

Cloned enzyme donor immunoassay（CEDIA）　克隆酶供体免疫分析

Microparticle enzyme immunoassay（MEIA）　微粒子酶免疫分析

Particle-enhanced turbidimetric inhibition immunoassay（PETINIA）
颗粒增强浊度抑制免疫分析法

Chemiluminescent microparticle immunoassay（CMIA）　化学发光微粒免疫分析

Antibody-conjugated magnetic immunoassay（ACMIA）　抗体标记磁性免疫分析

Enzyme-linked immunosorbent assay（ELISA）　酶联免疫吸附试验

2　*Readings*

Therapeutic drug monitoring（TDM）is the measurement of blood drug concentration to aid in optimizing drug therapy for patient care. It is based on that the therapeutic effect of drugs correlates better with their blood concentration than with the administered dose. However, only certain kinds of drugs need TDM, and there are some criteria to decide which drugs should be monitored. The trough concentration（C_0）, peak concentration and limited sampling strategies are the commonly-used clinical TDM strategies. The main methods for TDM are immunoassay and chromatographic. And the samples are serum, plasma, whole blood, saliva, and so on.

TDM is applied in many clinical areas.

2. 1   Introduction

Therapeutic drug monitoring (TDM) is the management of a patient's drug regimen based on the serum, plasma, or whole blood concentration of a drug. The International Association of Therapeutic Drug Monitoring & Clinical Toxicology has adopted the following definition: "Therapeutic drug monitoring (TDM) is defined as the measurement made in the laboratory of a parameter that, with appropriate interpretation, will directly influence prescribing procedures. Commonly, the measurement is in a biological matrix of a prescribed xenobiotic, but it may also be of an endogenous compound prescribed as replacement therapy in an individual who is physiologically or pathologically deficient in that compound. "

The great majority of drugs are managed in a standard way: they are dosed on a unit per body mass (e. g. mg/kg) basis, and then the dosage is adjusted based on the clinical response empirically assessed by a physician. This is often described as "titration to clinical effect". For a small subset of drugs, the clinical effects (pharmacodynamics) can be assessed objectively— for instance, antihypertensive drugs and blood pressure measurement, Coumadin and assessment of coagulation via international normalized ratio measurement, or statin drugs and blood lipid levels. For an even smaller subset of drugs, the pharmacokinetic-pharmacodynamic relationship is not predictable from the dose, and the pharmacokinetics is highly variable between individuals. For these drugs, management can be particularly challenging and for these drugs, TDM is the most effective. TDM is valuable when the drug has a narrow therapeutic index and toxicity which may be encountered at a concentration slightly above the upper end of the therapeutic range. There are approximately 6000 prescription and nonprescription (over-the-counter) drugs available for clinical use, but most of them have a wide therapeutic index and do not require routine TDM. 20 – 26 drugs are routinely monitored in clinical laboratories, whereas there are an additional 25 – 30 drugs that may benefit from TDM.

What kind of drugs needs TDM? There are several criteria: (1) the relationship between drug blood concentration and clinical or toxic effect must be well-defined, (2) the drugs must have a narrow therapeutic index (the difference between the minimum effective concentration and the toxic concentration), (3) the relationship between the drug dose and drug concentration in the blood must be highly variable and/or not predictable, (4) there should be serious consequences for under-or over-dosing, (5) the result of TDM testing must be interpretable and actionable, and there should be an effect on clinical outcomes, (6) there are accurate, reliable and applicable methods for drug concentration detection.

2. 2   Strategies for TDM

Since drugs are xenobiotics and the concentrations vary with time, blood sampling is critical to provide a correct interpretation of the drug exposure. It is generally accepted that the best marker of total drug exposure (efficacy or toxicity) is the full area under the concentration-time curve (AUC). However, the determination of full AUC is rather difficult to be obtained clinically both for ethical and nursing reasons due to the high number of blood specimens necessary and the long duration of time.

In clinical practice, TDM is performed by a collection of a blood sample at a known time point relative to administration of the last (or next) dose. For most of the drugs, the trough concentration (C_0) is used as the reference concentration. For some drugs, it is advisable to evaluate both the C_0 and the peak concentration to enable the determination of a possible accumulation and optimal efficacy. For mycophendic acid (MPA), limited sampling strategies (LSSs) from multiple concentration-time points (usually no more than 4-time points) are recommended in clinical practice. Multiple samples are collected for MPA concentration detection in the hours following drug intake and the AUC is estimated by computing the results by trapezoidal rule, multiple linear regressions, or Bayesian estimation.

Usually, Serum or plasma is used for TDM except for immunosuppressive drugs such as cyclosporine, tacrolimus, sirolimus, and everolimus, whose TDM is conducted using whole blood. During continuous therapy, blood should be obtained when a steady state has been reached, i. e. , after the administration of a constant dose for at least 5 times the half-life of the drug. Sampling should be performed according to the clinical situation either at the time of peak serum concentration and/or immediately before administration of the next dose (trough concentration). The timing of blood sampling to measure trough and peak concentrations is important for drugs with a narrow therapeutic range and a short half-life, e. g. theophylline, gentamicin, and certain antiarrhythmic agents. With some medications, e. g. phenytoin and phenobarbital, the timing of blood sampling is not critical since the differences between trough and peak serum concentrations are relatively small once the steady state has reached. After intravenous drug administration, the collection of the blood sampling has to be performed after the initial distribution phase has been completed. With most drugs, this will be achieved after 1 – 2h, with digoxin and digitoxin after 6 – 8h.

2. 3　Methods of determination

Different types of assays are used in clinical laboratories for TDM. The main methods are immunoassay and chromatographic methods.

2. 3. 1　Immunoassay for TDM

Most TDM testing is now performed by immunoassays in which specimens (serum or plasma) can be used without any pretreatment, and they are running on fully automated, continuous, and random accessed systems. For analysis of immunosuppressants (except mycophenolic acid) using whole blood specimen, a pretreatment phase may be required. The immunoassays require very small amounts of sample, and reagents are stored in the analyzer and most analyzers have stored calibration curves in the system.

In immunoassays, the analyte is detected by its binding with a specific molecule, which in most cases is an analyte-specific antibody (or a pair of specific antibodies). For assay design, there are two formats of immunoassays: competition-based and immunometric (commonly referred to as "sandwich"). Competition-based immunoassay is the method of choice for the analytes with small molecular weight, requiring a single analyte-specific antibody. In contrast, sandwich immunoassays are mostly used for analytes with larger molecular weight, such as proteins or peptides, and use two different specific antibodies. Because most TDM immunoassays involve analytes of small molecular size, the competition-based format is more commonly employed. In this format, the analyte molecules in the specimen compete with analyte (or its analogs) labeled with a suitable tag provided in the reagent, for a limited number of binding sites provided by an analyte-specific antibody (also provided in the reagent). Thus, in these types of assays, the higher the analyte concentration in the sample, the lower amount of label that can bind to the antibody to form the conjugate. If the bound label provides the signal, which in turn is used to calculate the analyte concentration in the sample, the analyte concentration in the specimen is inversely proportional to the signal produced. If the free label provides the signal, then the signal produced is proportional to the analyte concentration. The signal is mostly optical absorbance, fluorescence, or chemiluminescence. There are several variations in this basic format. The assay can be homogeneous or heterogeneous. In the former, the bound label has different properties from the free label, and no separation between the bound and free labels is needed before measuring the signal. In a heterogeneous assay format, the bound label must be separated from the free label. Commonly used formats of immunoassays in TDM include fluorescence polarization immunoassay (FPIA), enzyme-multiplied immunoassay technique (EMIT), cloned enzyme donor immunoassay (CEDIA), microparticle enzyme immunoassay (MEIA), particle-enhanced turbidimetric inhibition immunoassay (PETINIA), chemiluminescent microparticle immunoassay (CMIA), antibody-conjugated magnetic immunoassay (ACMIA) and enzyme-linked immunosorbent assay (ELISA).

Although the immunoassay methods are now widely used, there are significant limitations. Antibody specificity is the major concern about immunoassay. Many endogenous metabolites of the analyte (drug) may have a very similar structural recognition motif to the analyte. There may also be other molecules unrelated to the analyte but producing comparable recognition motif as the analyte. These molecules are generally called cross-reactants. When presenting in the sample, these molecules may produce both positive and negative interference in the relevant immunoassay. Other components in a specimen, such as bilirubin, hemoglobin, or lipid, may interfere in the immunoassay by interfering with the assay signal, thus producing incorrect results. The third type of immunoassay interference involves endogenous human antibodies in the specimen, which may interfere with components of the assay reagent such as the assay antibodies or the antigen labels. Such interference includes the interference from heterophilic antibodies or various human anti-animal antibodies. However, interference of heterophilic antibody in immunoassays used for TDM is reported rarely.

Immunoassays are not commercially available for all drugs currently monitored in clinical practice, for example, antiretroviral agents. For monitoring such drugs, sophisticated techniques such as high-performance liquid chromatography combined with tandem mass spectrometry (HPLC-MS/MS) are usually used. In general, chromatography-based methods (including LC-MS/MS) for TDM are superior approaches compared to immunoassays because such methods are relatively free from interferences. For immunosuppressants where immunoassays are commercially available, chromatographic methods, particularly LC-MS/MS methods, are considered as the "gold standard" due to significant metabolite cross-reactivity in immunoassays for the parent drug.

2.3.2 LC-MS/MS for TDM

Conventional immunoassays may lack the required sensitivity and specificity for accurate measurement of therapeutic drugs, and as a result, liquid chromatographic (LC) methods combined with mass spectrometry (referred to as LC-MS and LC-MS/MS) were initially developed in clinical laboratories. Such analytical platforms have been implemented in both clinical and reference laboratory settings for nearly two decades. The ability of LC to separate individual compounds from other drugs and metabolites present in the biological matrix, combined with selective MS techniques to provide further mass-based delineation, has resulted in its superior sensitivity and specificity over immunoassays. As a result, for certain drugs, such as immunosuppressants, LC-MS and LC-MS/MS methodologies are preferred over immunoassays for TDM. In addition, the simultaneous measurement of multiple drugs within a single specimen source using an LC-MS based-platform has decreased the need for higher sample volumes for carrying out various individual tests, and it may even provide improvements on turnaround times (TATs). Traditionally, TDM measurements have been carried out in blood matrix such as plasma or serum; drug quantification in tissue biopsies, dried blood spots, and oral fluid are becoming potential alternatives for TDM measurements. LC-MS platforms provide the advantage of drug quantification in such matrices.

However, LC-MS methods are also associated with several limitations in the clinical laboratory setting. Currently, LC-MS and LC-MS/MS assays are laboratory-developed tests (LDTs) that are not subjected to premarket approval processes and strict supervisions. At the same time, LC-MS and LC-MS/MS assays may also exhibit interlaboratory variability that could potentially impact TDM measurements in patient populations that require prolonged follow-up from multiple health care settings. Furthermore, the presence of certain interfering substances in specimen samples such as salts and phospholipids can cause matrix effects that may result in significant fluctuations during compound ionization. Due to the high technical expertise required for its operation, there is also a demand for highly skilled personnel. The initial high installation costs, especially for implementation in small-and medium-scale laboratories, the time investment for personnel training and method validation, and integration into laboratory workflow for maximum throughput and reduced TAT are some of the factors that require careful considerations before incorporating LC-MS or LC-MS/MS-based platforms into the clinical laboratory.

Despite the mentioned limitations, LC-MS and LC-MS/MS-based assays are utilized in cases in which traditional immunoassays cannot be implemented. In addition, with combinatorial drug therapies being recommended as first-line treatments for antiretroviral agents, immunosuppressive drugs, and anticonvulsants, the use of multiplexed LC-MS assays provides analytical measurements with diminished volume requirements and TAT. In the past two decades, LC combined with MS has shown tremendous potential for its implementation in clinical laboratories in the field of TDM. Enhanced sensitivity, specificity, precision and accuracy have been favorable factors for its use, whereas matrix effects, higher interlaboratory variability, and increased physical labor have been trade-offs. With the growing technological advancements in LC and MS instrumentations, there is a promising hope that the LC-MS platforms will serve the field of patient health care with high quality and timely contributions.

2.4   Clinical application

Drugs are being under-dosed or over-dosed more frequently than generally assumed. The pharmacological response of a patient to a given dosage regimen is determined by several factors, including patient compliance, bioavailability, serum (or whole blood) drug level, rate of elimination, and the access of the drug to the receptor site as well as the receptor sensitivity. TDM is very useful when there is a good correlation between serum or whole blood drug concentration and the clinical response.

The primary function of TDM is to guide reasonable adjustment of the drug dose. Following drug ingestion or administration to a patient, absorption, distribution, metabolism, elimination, as well as therapeutic efficacy may be variable. Collection of blood for drug analysis can be used to determine if the patient is within a target therapeutic window or has subtherapeutic or toxic drug concentrations. Based on drug concentrations, dose adjustments may be made to improve treatment efficacy (Figure 8 − 1).

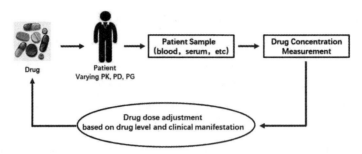

Figure 8 - 1   The process of therapeutic drug monitoring (TDM).

At the same time, there are other applications of TDM results. For example, TDM in antiretroviral management in patients with HIV is not necessary for the optimization of dose. However, it is vitally important to confirm adherence to the prescribed drug regimen in the context of increasing viral loads and apparent therapeutic failure. The TDM results can be used to assist in the determination of whether the patient has developed viral resistance to the prescribed drugs or whether the patient has simply stopped taking the drugs. Another question that can be answered is whether the drug is being absorbed in all. For instance, gastrointestinal (GI) inflammation could prevent drugs administered orally from entering the circulation. It is important to remember that TDM is a tool for assessing the clinical presentation of the patient.

Although TDM is more common for drugs used in treating a chronic illness (e. g. epilepsy and cardiac dysfunction), certain antibiotics (e. g. vancomycin and aminoglycosides) are routinely monitored in treating an acute life-threatening infection due to the inherent toxicity of these drugs, mainly nephrotoxicity and ototoxicity.

The followings are the clinical areas in which TDM is a routine practice.

2.4.1   Antiepileptic drugs

For the treatment of epilepsy, TDM has significant value because the antiepileptic drugs act on the central nervous system (CNS) to treat the seizures, but they also can cause toxic CNS effects. In some cases, the drugs can cause seizures, making it difficult to differentiate subtherapeutic effects from toxic effects. TDM is useful to quickly determine whether drug concentration is too low or too high upon initiation of therapy. In addition, once a baseline concentration has been established for patients on chronic therapy, blood levels can be used to investigate the loss of seizure control or unexpected toxicity in a stable patient. TDM is recommended for these classical antiepileptic drugs: phenytoin, fosphenytoin (prodrug for phenytoin), carbamazepine, primidone, phenobarbital, valproic acid, and newer generation antiepileptic drugs: lamotrigine, levetiracetam, gabapentin and oxcarbazepine (MHC, a biologically active metabolite is analyzed).

2.4.2   Immunosuppressive drugs

Organ transplantation is an extremely complex medical procedure, to suppress rejection and increase the survival rate of transplantation, immunosuppressive drugs must be used in the remainder of patients' life. Management of these powerful drugs requires a balance of ensuring enough drug exposure to prevent rejection while keeping the concentration of the drug low enough to avoid toxic effects. TDM is an essential tool in the process, allowing rapid titration of blood concentrations of the drug to maximize immunosuppression and avoid acute rejection while minimizing adverse events from exposure to the drugs. Tacrolimus, cyclosporine A, sirolimus, everolimus and mycophenolic acid (MPA) are routine targets of TDM in clinical practice.

2.4.3　Antiarrhythmic drugs

Historically in cardiology, certain therapeutic agents have been used to control arrhythmia in patients with abnormal heart physiology. However, these historic therapeutic agents display two important tendencies. First, each of the agents demonstrates significant pharmacokinetic variability. Second, although these agents can control arrhythmia when the dose is optimized, they can also cause arrhythmia when concentrations in blood are too high. Based on these characteristics, it is recognized that TDM is a pivotal tool in the optimal management of these agents. TDM is recommended for procainamide, lidocaine, lidocaine, and digoxin.

2.4.4　Antipsychotic drugs

In the treatment of psychiatric disorders such as depression or schizophrenia, pharmacotherapy is commonly managed by titration to clinical effect. This approach is taken because of the lack of robust relationship between the dose administered (or blood concentration) and the clinical response to therapy. In addition, it is difficult to investigate these relationships because the clinical endpoint of response is somewhat subjective and can vary based on the variability of how the patients communicate their experience and the way the clinicians perceive their interaction with the patients. However, for some drugs, the adverse effects can be objectively measured and correlated with the blood concentration of the drug. In these cases, TDM can be a useful tool for patient management, such as lithium and tricyclic antidepressants (including amitriptyline, nortriptyline, imipramine, desipramine, and clomipramine).

2.4.5　Antibiotics and antifungal drugs

In the treatment of infectious diseases, the biological activity of the drug is directed against the microorganism responsible for the infection and not influencing the host (the person taking the drug). As such, the therapeutic index is quite wide, and although many of the drugs have significant pharmacokinetic variability and it is important to have the drug concentration higher than the minimal effective concentration (MIC) for eradication of the microorganism, the lack of toxic effects against the host allows for a high dose relative to the MIC to ensure sufficient blood concentrations for microbicidal effect. However, some antimicrobial drugs do have both significant pharmacokinetic variability and significant clinical toxicity for the host. In these cases, TDM is a valuable tool for the management of the drugs, for example, aminoglycoside antibiotics (gentamicin, tobramycin and amikacin), vancomycin, voriconazole, posaconazole, and so on.

2.4.6 Anti-tumor drugs

In the treatment of cancer, most drugs are dosed based on body surface area normalization, and then the patients are monitored for significant toxicity or clinical effect—this is similar to the classic titrate to clinical effect paradigm. However, in cancer treatment, the additional parameter of maximum tolerated dose (MTD) must be considered. Because the drugs are known to be toxic (they are cytotoxic drugs after all), part of the clinical trials during drug development involve assessment of dose-limiting toxicity relative to the administered dose in a small number of patients to determine the maximum amount of drug that should be given. When patients are receiving the MTD and not exhibiting symptoms of toxicity, treatment is continued without dose adjustment until it is determined whether the treatment is affecting cancer. However, it is important to note that many chemotherapy drugs have significant pharmacokinetic variability so that when MTD is given to the patient and no toxic effects are observed, it is not certain that the patient is getting the correct dose; it may be that the patient is getting less drug than needed (or that he or she can tolerate). Based on this, some have advocated for the concept of maximum tolerated exposure, which would require blood concentration measurements. TDM is not a routine practice in the management of chemotherapy. Methotrexate and busulfan are the exception. For these two drugs, TDM is recommended to ensure the therapeutic effect and avoid toxicity in the treatment of malignancy.

TDM is now a mature field in laboratory medicine, with several well-established applications and a history of almost 50 years, but with recent advances in healthcare information systems and technologies for rapid measurement of drug concentrations in biological matrices, the real advances to optimize TDM practices for improving patient outcomes are just beginning.

3 Discussion

(1) What is TDM?

(2) Why TDM is needed in clinical practice? Is TDM necessary for all drugs?

(3) How to do clinical TDM (sample type, sample collection and analytical method)?

Resources and references

[1] CLARKE W, DASGUPTA A. Clinical challenges in therapeutic drug monitoring [M]. Amsterdam: Elsevier, 2016.

[2] DASGUPTA A. Therapeutic drug monitoring [M]. Amsterdam: Elsevier, 2012.

[3] GREBE S K, SINGH R J. LC-MS/MS in the clinical laboratory—where to from here? [J]. Clin Biochem Rev, 2011, 32 (1): 5 - 31.

[4] MARZINKE MA, CLARKE W. Laboratory developed tests in the clinical laboratory: challenges for implementation [J]. Bioanalysis, 2015, 7 (15): 1817 - 1820.

[5] CHRISTIANS U, VINKS A A, LANGMAN L J, et al. Impact of laboratory practices on interlaboratory variability in therapeutic drug monitoring of immunosuppressive drugs [J]. Ther Drug Monit, 2015, 37 (6): 718 - 724.

[6] ADAWAY J E, KEEVIL B G. Therapeutic drug monitoring and LC-MS/MS [J]. J Chromatogr B Analyt Technol Biomed Life Sci, 2012, 883 - 884.

（白杨娟）

CHAPTER 9
CELLULAR IMMUNITY AND LABORATORY ASSAYS

1 *Words and phrases*

Innate immunity　固有免疫（天然免疫）

Adaptive immunity　适应性免疫（获得性免疫）

Phagocyte/Phagocytic cell　吞噬细胞

Macrophage　巨噬细胞

Complement system　补体系统

Cytokine　细胞因子

Chemokine　趋化因子

Chemotaxis　趋化性

Humoral　体液的

Immunoglobulin　免疫球蛋白

Antigen-presenting cell（APC）　抗原提呈细胞

Dendritic cell　树突状细胞

Cytotoxic　细胞毒性的

Perforin　穿孔素

Granzyme　颗粒酶

Regulatory T cell（Treg cell）　调节性 T 细胞

Helper T cell（Th cell）　辅助性 T 细胞

T follicular helper cell（Tfh cell）　滤泡辅助 T 细胞

Parasite　寄生虫

Intestinal helminth　肠蠕虫

Proinflammatory　前炎症的

Apoptosis　凋亡

Hematopoietic　造血的

Nonlymphoid　非淋巴样的

Mucosal　黏膜的

Inducible costimulator　可诱导共刺激分子

Flow cytometry（FCM）　流式细胞术

Immunofluorescence　免疫荧光

Forward scatter（FS）　前向散射（光）

Side scatter（SS）　侧向散射（光）

Fluorescence（FL）　荧光

Nuclear contour　核轮廓

Granularity　粒度

Immunocompetence　免疫能力

Mitogenic　有丝分裂的

Concanavalin A（Con A）　伴刀豆球蛋白 A，伴刀豆凝集素 A

Phytohemagglutinin（PHA）　植物血凝素

Immunogen　免疫原

Antigen　抗原

Antibody　抗体

Liquid scintillation counter　液体闪烁计数器

Carboxyfluorescein diacetate succinimidyl ester（CFSE）
羧基荧光素二乙酸琥珀酰亚胺酯

Permeant　渗透的

Esterase　酯酶

Acetate group　乙酸基团

Succinimidyl ester　琥珀酰亚胺酯

Free amine　游离胺

Adduct　加合物

Mixed lymphocyte culture　混合淋巴细胞培养

Cell-mediated lysis assay　细胞介导的溶细胞分析

Enzyme-linked immunosorbent spot assay（ELISPOT）　酶联免疫吸附斑点试验

Enzyme-linked immunosorbent assay（ELISA）　酶联免疫吸附试验

Chromium　铬

Supernatant　上清液

Tritium-labeled thymidine　氚标记胸苷

Fluorescein　荧光素

2 *Readings*

2.1 Introduction

2.1.1 Immunity

Immunity is a process or a series of responses to protect bodies from all kinds of diseases, usually from infectious diseases. Immune responses against microbes or foreign materials include early reactions of innate immunity and the later responses of adaptive immunity. Innate immunity consists of cellular and biochemical defense mechanism against microbes, which mainly includes physical and chemical barriers, phagocytic cells (such as neutrophils, macrophages) and NK cells, complement system, as well as cytokines and chemokines. Adaptive immunity is later immune responses to foreign organisms with more specificity and immune memory, which is subdivided into two types, humoral immunity, and cellular immunity. Humoral immunity is mediated by antibodies or immunoglobulins produced by B cells or plasma cells, and is the principal immune response by antibodies binding to extracellular microbes and their toxins so as to eliminate them. However for intracellular microbes, such as viruses and some bacteria, circulating antibodies cannot be accessible to bind them, and cellular immunity mediated by T cells is necessary to eliminate infected cells and intracellular microbes. Here we will focus on the conception of cellular immunity and its analysis methods.

2.1.2 Cellular immunity

Cellular immunity, also called cell-mediated immunity, is one type of adaptive immunity, which is mediated by many types of T cells to respond to a specific challenge, usually a foreign organism or material. Actually, immune system works as a whole, the interactions among different cells are required in innate and adaptive immunity. Antigen-presenting cells (APC) in innate immunity, such as dendritic cells and macrophages, take part in the activation of lymphocytes in adaptive immunity. The interaction between helper T cells and B cells induces the activation of B cells. In addition to the direct cell-contact manner, cytokines and chemokines produced by all kinds of immune cells also play a vital role in cell communication and immune responses.

In cellular immunity, different types of T cells can be categorized into two main groups, $CD4^+$ T cells, and $CD8^+$ T cells. Generally, $CD4^+$ T cells, also called helper T cells (Ths), are cytokine-secreting cells, mainly activate other T cells or B cells, and $CD8^+$ T cells are cytotoxic T lymphocytes (CTL), mainly kill the infected cells by negative signals way or granule proteins, especially perforin and granzymes. $CD4^+$ T cells are the core cells to take part in regulating different cells (such as B cells, macrophages, and effector T cells) through direct cell contact and/or cytokine signaling. According to the classical cytokine secretion pattern, $CD4^+$ T cells have been classified into Th1 cells and Th2 cells. The Th1 subset mainly secretes interleukin-2 (IL-2), interleukin-12 (IL-12), tumor necrosis factor-α (TNF-α) and interferon-γ (IFN-γ), which promote their interaction with neutrophils or macrophages and mediate cytotoxicity and local inflammatory reactions. The Th2 subset produces interleukin-4 (IL-4), interleukin-5 (IL-5), interleukin-6 (IL-6), and interleukin-10 (IL-10), which mainly activate B cells and induce humoral immunity.

Recently more different subtypes of $CD4^+$ T cells have been identified (Figure 9 – 1), which are characterized by surface CD4 positive and producing different sets of cytokines and having different biological functions. Th9, Th17, Th22, Th25, regulatory T cells (Tregs), and T follicular helper (Tfh) cells are separate subtypes from Th1 and Th2 cells, and they have been demonstrated to be critical in the pathogenesis of autoimmune diseases, inflammation and tumor. Th9 cells mainly producing interleukin-9 (IL-9) play a vital role in protecting against extracellular parasites and intestinal helminth infections, and they are also proinflammatory cells that could stimulate proliferation and inhibit apoptosis of hematopoietic cells and activate Th17 cells. Th17 cells mainly secreting interleukin-17A (IL-17A), interleukin-17F (IL-17F), and interleukin-22 (IL-22), as one of the key inflammatory cells, take part in anti-infection, the pathogenesis and processing of autoimmune diseases, and transplant rejection. Th22 cells mainly produce IL-22, interleukin-13 (IL-13), fibroblast growth factor, chemokine ligand 15 (CCL15), chemokine ligand 17 (CCL17), and tumor necrosis factor-α (TNF-α), and participate in wound repair and in protection against bacterial, viral, and fungal infections at epithelial surfaces of the skin and gastrointestinal tract. Th25 cells mainly producing interleukin-25 (IL-25), IL-4, IL-5, and IL-13 can activate nonlymphoid cells to secret effector cytokines in response to extracellular pathogens, especially function in mucosal immunity. Tregs are one type of important immunosuppressive or tolerance cells, which are characterized by surface $CD4^+$, $CD25^+$, $CD127^-$ and intracellular transcription factor forkhead box P3 (FOXP3)$^+$. They have two ways to play an immunosuppressive role, including cell-cell contact and cytokines-mediated suppressing function. Negative signal molecules on Tregs, such as programmed cell death protein-1 (PD-1), CD152, and anti-inflammatory cytokines, such as IL-10, interleukin-35 (IL-35) and transforming growth factor-β (TGF-β), are both necessary to the suppressive role of Tregs. Tfh cells, one type of professional B cell helper cells, are mainly localized in B cell follicle and germinal center of lymph node, and assist B cells activation and antibodies production. Until now Tfh cells are considered as one kind of critical T cell subset to participate in antibodies class-switch and high-affinity antibodies producing. They are characterized by surface $CD4^+$, C-X-C chemokine receptor 5 (CXCR 5)$^+$, inducible costimulator (ICOS)$^+$ and CD40 ligand (CD40L), intracellular B cell CLL/lymphoma 6 (Bcl 6)$^+$, and guide B cells into germinal centers by chemotaxis mediated by CXCR5 signaling, as well as play a role in immunoglobulins production through interleukin-21 (IL-21).

With the new methods and technology developing, more and more T cell subsets will be defined according to intra-and extra-cellular proteins and genes. Whatever kind of T cell subsets is important to take part in effector cells generation and activation in innate or adaptive immunity.

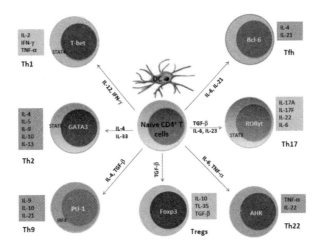

Figure 9 - 1   Differentiation of naive CD4 $^+$ T cells into CD4 $^+$ T cell subsets. (**see Appendix Figure 8**)

The picture is derived from Liu Z, Fan H, Jiang S. CD4 (+) T-cell subsets in transplantation [J]. Immunol Rev. 2013 Mar; 252 (1): 183 - 191.

2. 2   Laboratory assays for the function of cellular immunity

Cellular immunity mainly refers to different subtypes of T cells, such as Th1, Th2, Th17, Tregs, and Tfh cells. T lymphocyte assays in clinical laboratory generally include lymphocyte subsets percentage or count assay and function assay. Different assays are done based on different clinical significance, testing principles, and instruments.

2. 2. 1   Lymphocyte count assay

Lymphocyte subsets percentage or count assay is done according to lymphocyte surface or intracellular specific antigens or proteins as markers to define some type of lymphocytes. And the test methods consist of manual work with microscopic tests (been obsoleted) and flow cytometry with fluorescence-labeled antibodies. Here we will focus on flow cytometry used to detect lymphocyte subsets percentage or count.

Flow cytometry (FCM) is a very powerful and useful tool to detect single-cell characteristics, including identifying cell types, counting cell numbers and analyzing cell function. Flow cytometer, an instrument based on flow cytometry principle, combines a flow cell apparatus and complex optical system with direct or indirect immunofluorescence-labeled antibodies to specifically identify cell surface or intracellular antigens. Multi-parameters including forward scatter (FS), side scatter (SS), and several fluorescences (FL) can identify cell type and demonstrate cell function. The intensity of FS correlates with cell size; the intensity of SS correlates with cell complexity, such as nuclear contour, granularity. The intensity of FL reflects the number of antigens with a corresponding fluorescence tag. For example, lymphocytes can easily be distinguished from neutrophils by comparing FS, SS or CD45 expression. (Figure 9 − 2A, B) Cell surface markers (such as CD antigens) are associated with different subtypes, stages of cell development. For example, CD3 is a marker for T cells, and CD19 or CD20 is the specific marker for B cells. How to phenotype T cells is mainly based on surface CD3, CD4 and CD8 expression. In Figure 9 − 2 it shows that CD45 $^+$ cells are lymphocytes, and CD3 $^+$ lymphocytes are T cells, CD3 $^+$ CD4 $^+$ T cells are classically called helper T cells, CD3 $^+$ CD8 $^+$ T cells are generally called cytotoxic T cells. Once cell types can be identified, the percentage or numbers of target cells could be easily counted.

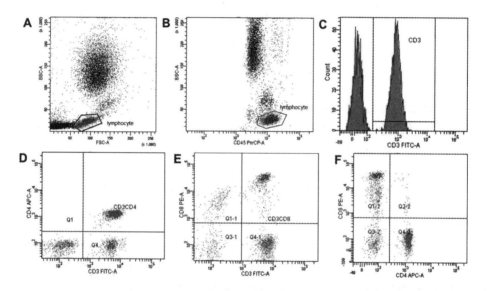

Figure 9 − 2 Flow cytometry analysis for peripheral T cells phenotype. (see Appendix Figure 9)

A. It shows diverse cell types in a scatter graph with SS vs. FS. B. It shows diverse cell types in a scatter graph with SS vs. CD45. C. CD3 $^+$ cells expression gated on lymphocytes. D. CD3 $^+$ CD4 $^+$ T cells expression gated on lymphocytes. E. CD3 $^+$ CD8 $^+$ T cells expression gated on lymphocytes. F. Scatter graph with CD8 vs. CD4 to show CD8 $^+$ cells and CD4 $^+$ cells expression gated on lymphocytes.

2.2.2 Lymphocyte function assay

Not only lymphocyte numbers but also their function are both important to the effect of cellular immunity. Lymphocyte numbers could be influenced by its proliferation competence, and lymphocyte proliferation assay could directly reflect the reaction of cells to immune stimulators. Lymphocyte function assay includes T-cell function assay and B-cell function assay. Assays designed to detect antibodies produced by B cells are mainly used to assess humoral immunocompetence. Because this chapter focuses on cellular immunity that mainly refers to T lymphocytes, here we will pay attention to T-cell function assay. T-cell function assays generally measure T-cell proliferative responses, T-cell effector responses, and T-cell cytokine profiles.

2.2.3   T-cell proliferation assay

The assay is used to assess the proliferative responses of T cells to mitogenic stimuli or activation signals. Generally, stimuli to T cell proliferation and activation are concanavalin A (Con A) and phytohemagglutinin (PHA), as well as cell-activation-related signal molecules or their antibodies such as anti-CD3 and anti-CD28 antibodies or IL-2. In general, mitogen-stimulated lymphocyte activation and proliferation are polyclonal responses, and lymphocyte proliferation responses to immunogens are antigen-specific.

Proliferation analysis can be carried out in a static or dynamic method. Static analysis can quantify the cell cycle fraction of a given cell population. And dynamic analysis can demonstrate the absolute duration of the individual cell cycle phase and the regulation of cell proliferation under defined cell culture conditions. The magnitude of T cell proliferation can be measured by adding DNA or intracellular proteins-binding dyes to the medium during cell culture and then quantitating its incorporation into the DNA or its binding with intracellular proteins of dividing cells by liquid scintillation counter or flow cytometry. The general methods to detect cell proliferation include anti-BrdU technology, BrdU-Hoechst quenching technology, and carboxyfluorescein diacetate succinimidyl ester (CFSE) dying.

Static DNA analysis only shows a snapshot of the distribution of a cell population in a cell cycle phase. The size of the S phase fraction (SPF) is considered as a proxy for the proliferation activity of the cells of interest. The higher SPF the analysis shows, the stronger proliferation activity the population of interest has. However, only dynamic DNA analysis could demonstrate more detailed information about proliferation.

Dynamic proliferation analysis is far more informative than static cell cycle analysis, and enables investigation into the regulation of cell proliferation under defined conditions, as well as determines the momentary cell cycle distribution. Dynamic analysis with flow cytometry can calculate the distribution of cells according to a phase of the cell cycle, quantify the percentage of resting cells (G_0 phase cells), determine the absolute duration of the phases of the cell cycle, and retrace the replication history of individual cells.

CFSE, a fluorescein derivative, is cell-permeant and non-fluorescent. After CFSE permeates into the cell, cellular esterases can cleave acetate groups, and cleaved products become fluorescent and cell impermeant; succinimidyl ester binds to free amines. Finally, CFSE results in long lived fluorescent adducts. With cell proliferation and division, CFSE will be divided into the next generation cell population, in which the fluorescence intensity of CFSE is weakened to half of the undivided cells. With increasing proliferation, the fluorescence intensity of CFSE in divided cells gradually decreases. (Figure 9 - 3, Figure 9 - 4)

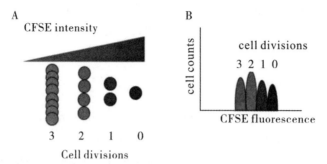

Figure 9 - 3   Schematic diagram of CFSE dying in cell proliferation. (see Appendix Figure 10)

A. it shows the fluorescence intensity of CFSE decreases with cell divisions. B. it shows the schematic diagram of CFSE analyzed in flow cytometry.

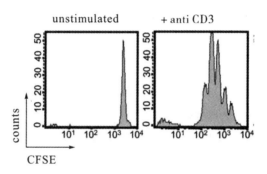

Figure 9 - 4   Flow cytometry histogram of CFSE dying for T cell proliferation analysis.
(see Appendix Figure 11)

The picture is derived from Schneider MA, Meingassner JG, Lipp M, et al. CCR7 is required for the in vivo function of CD4 $^+$ CD25 $^+$ regulatory T cells [J]. J Exp Med, 2007, 204 (4): 735 - 745.

2. 2. 4   T-cell effector responses assay

As we know effector T cells are mainly CD8 $^+$ T cells, which play a cytotoxic role in immune responses, especially for pathogens-infected cells, tumor cells, and non-self cells. Here we mainly introduce the methods to analyze the function of cytotoxicity of T cells.

Generally mixed lymphocyte culture (MLC) and cell-mediated lysis (CML) assay are used to measure the cytotoxic function of CD8 $^+$ T cells. In the assay, CD8 $^+$ T cells are incubated with labeled target cells expressing an antigen to which the CD8 $^+$ T cells have been sensitized that originate from an unrelated individual used as stimulatory cells in the culture. By quantitating the numbers of labeled target cells by microscope or flow cytometry or other methods the cytotoxic function of CD8 $^+$ T cells can be measured. Chromium release assay and Jam test are both classic tests for measuring CTL function.

2.2.5   Chromium release assay

In the assay radioactive chromium (^{51}Cr) labeled target cells incubates with effector cells for 4 – 6 hours. Due to the cytotoxic role of effector cells, the target cells are lysed by perforins and granzymes, then radioactive chromium is released into the supernatant, which can be detected by a counter. The more effective the lysis is, the higher the amount of chromium released is. Maximal chromium release is achieved by lysing all of the cells in a suitable detergent (for example Triton, a kind of surfactants). The efficacy of cell lysis is partially dependent on the ratio of effector cells to target cells and it can be determined using a simple formula. The disadvantage is that dead cells due to apoptosis are not correctly measured in the assay. (Figure 9 – 5)

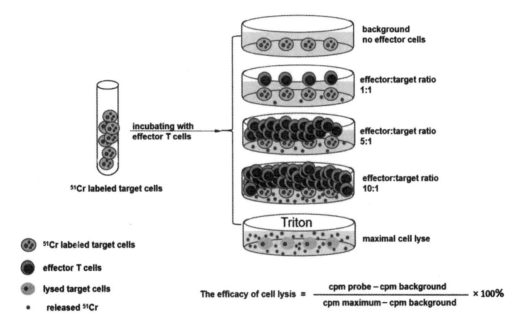

The efficacy of cell lysis $= \dfrac{\text{cpm probe} - \text{cpm background}}{\text{cpm maximum} - \text{cpm background}} \times 100\%$

Figure 9 – 5   Chromium release assay (one of the classical cytotoxicity assays).
(see Appendix Figure 12)

With the increase of effector T cells, more target cells lyse, and more ^{51}Cr are released. (cpm = counts per minute)

2.2.6   Jam test

As we know CTL can play a cytotoxic role with different ways including perforin, granzyme, and Fas-FasL pathway. The Fas-FasL pathway can induce apoptosis of Fas-expressing cells. Chromium release assay can't detect cells killed by apoptosis without cell lysis, so the assay often underestimates the killing efficacy of effector cells. Jam test measuring DNA concentration derived from different molecular-weights can correctly analyze the cytotoxicity of cells. Target cells were cultured in tritium-labeled thymidine coculture with effector cells. When apoptosis happens, labeled DNA is fragmented into tiny pieces. On the automated cell harvester, the low-molecular-weight DNA of apoptotic cells is removed with washing, and the high-molecular-weight DNA of intact cells is caught in the filter. The lysis rate can be calculated using the following formula.

$$\text{lysis rate} = \frac{\text{cpm without effector cell} - \text{cpm probe}}{\text{cpm without effector cell}} \times 100\%$$

Moreover, another assay to detect T cell effector responses is a test in vivo, for example, delayed-type hypersensitive. This assay measures the ability of helper T cells and APC cells to collaborate. This assay indicates that the immune responses of the body to an antigen previously exposed could induce a serial of immune reactions including Th cells activation, chemokines secreting, neutrophils transferring, and so on, to induce immune inflammation based on the interaction between innate and adaptive immune systems. In some clinical cases, this assay could help clinicians learn the immune status of patients or whether the patient has exposed to some key pathogens before.

2.2.7　T-cell cytokine-secreting function assay

After T cell activation different cytokines can be secreted from diverse T cells. Different cytokines secreted from different T cells determine the T cell subsets and their immune function. So T-cell cytokine profiles detection can help learning the immune status of the body. T cell cytokine profiles assays include quantitating cytokines in culture media by enzyme-linked immunosorbent assay (ELISA) and cytokines in T cells (intracellular cytokines) by flow cytometry or enzyme-linked immunosorbent spot assay (ELISPOT). Cytokine profiles in culture media just indicate the entire status for the cultured T cells, and intracellular cytokine profiles or cytokine ELISPOT analysis can reflet T cell subsets profile and their cytokine secretion function, which are more important to immune responses. Flow cytometry is a very useful method to analyze intracellular cytokine profiles, and can simultaneously detect multiple helper T cell subsets which are characterized by relatively specific and diverse cytokines.

2.2.8　Intracellular cytokine assay (T-cell cytokine profile assay)

T cells are incubated with mitogen and Golgi stop or Brefeldin A to induce T cells to produce cytokines and inhibit the extrusion of cytokines. Then they are stained with fluorescence-labeled antibodies to T cells surface antigens and intracellular cytokines. These cells can be detected with multicolor flow cytometer to identify CD4 $^+$ or CD8 $^+$ T cells and their cytokine patterns at the single-cell level. Intracellular cytokine assay with flow cytometry is a high throughput method, and combining with absolute count assay, it can provide cell count of specific cytokine-secreting cells. (Figure 9 − 6)

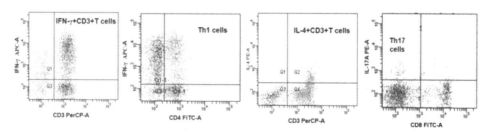

Figure 9 − 6   FCM scatter diagram to analyze intracellular cytokines expression in T cell subsets.
(see Appendix Figure 13)

IFN-γ $^+$ CD4 $^+$ T cells are defined as Th1 cells. IL-17A $^+$ CD4 $^+$ T cells are defined as Th17 cells.

2. 2. 9   Cytokine-secreting cells assay

ELISPOT is a common method to detect the frequency of antigen-specific T cells or T cells with specific cytokine-secreting function. Firstly, T cells incubates with antigen and APC in a well coated with specific antibodies against the target cytokine for 24 or 48 hours. After stimulation with antigens in the well, cytokines secreted by T cells are captured by membrane-bound antibodies on the spot. After incubation, the cells are removed by washing, and second enzyme-labeled antibodies against cytokines can bind the specific cytokine secreted by T cells. Finally, calculating the stained spots can indicate the frequency of cytokine-producing cells, which is expressed as the number of spot-forming cells (SFC) per 100000 cells. (Figure 9 − 7 and Figure 9 − 8)

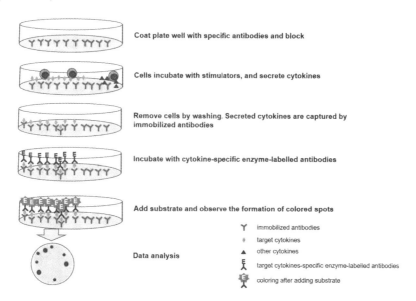

Figure 9 − 7   ELISPOT assay procedures. (see Appendix Figure 14)

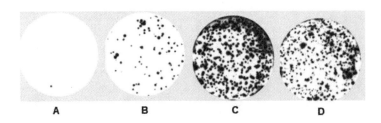

Figure 9 – 8   ELISOPT results to analyze the activities of T cells to secrete IFN-γ after stimulation.
(see Appendix Figure 15)

A. Only T cells are cultured in medium as the control group. B. CD8 $^+$ T cells are stimulated with a peptide pool consisting of 32 peptides of influenza A virus (Flu), cytomegalovirus (CMV) and Epstein-Barr virus (EBV) epitopes. C. CD4 $^+$ T cells are stimulated with staphylococcal enterotoxin B. D. T cells are stimulated with PHA as the positive control.

2. 2. 10   Cytokine-secreting cells isolation assay

Firstly, apply bispecific antibodies to capture activated T cells, which is characterized by CD45 or CD3, then bispecific antibodies can bind some specific cytokines secreted by the captured T cells, and second fluorescence-labeled antibodies bind with captured cytokines. Finally, they are isolated in FACS sorter or in a magnetic field (MACS) with the aid of iron-conjugated antibodies. This method could acquire the intact cell which has the specific cytokine-secreting function for further analysis.

Cellular immunity, as a critical part of adaptive immunity, takes part in all immune responses in infectious diseases, autoimmune disease, and transplantation immune, etc. T lymphocytes, as the major immune cells in cellular immunity, not only play a key supporting role in activating effector T cells, B cells and NK cells through secreting cytokines or in cell-contact manner, but also have an important effective role, such as cytotoxicity. Until now many technologies and assays, such as ELISA, ELISPOT, and flow cytometry, have been developed to count T cell subsets and analyze T lymphocytes' immune functions. In vitro determining T cells number and function is necessary to learn the status of cellular immunity of patients and helpful for clinicians to make a diagnosis or evaluate the effects of therapy, especially biotherapy.

3   Discussion

A male patient, 65 years old, felt fatigued and had a light fever with headache and cough for almost two weeks. RBC, PLT were both in the normal range, and WBC was $3.2 \times 10^9/L$, and lymphocytes percentage was 44%, liver function and renal function were both normal. After physical examination, enlarged lymph nodes were palpable in the anterior and posterior cervical and inguinal areas. The chest CT scan showed that there was some inflammation in the lung. The EBV and CMV DNA quantitation indicated he had EBV and CMV infection. Peripheral T cells subset percentage showed T cells were 67% , CD4$^+$T cells were 10% and CD8$^+$T cells were 52% .

(1) What can the above medical history and laboratory results indicate?

(2) Which test or assay do you think to do for further diagnosis?

(3) How do you think to evaluate T cells function?

(4) What methods can be used to determine cytokine-secreting function of T cells? And describe them in detail.

References and resources

[1] STROBER W, GOTTESMAN S R S. Immunology: clinical case studies and disease pathophysiology [M]. New Jersey: A John Wiley & Sons, Inc. , 2009.

[2] ABBAS A K, LICHTMAN A H, PILLAI S. Cellular and molecular immunology [M]. 9th edition. Philadelphia: Elsevier Inc. , 2018.

[3] ROITT I, BROSTOFF J, Male D. Immunology [M]. 6th ed. London: Mosby, 2001.

[4] SACK U, TÁRNOK A, ROTHE G. Cellular diagnostics: basic principle, methods and clinical application of flow cytometry [M]. Basel: Karger Medical and Scientific Publishers, 2009.

[5] CAZA T, LANDAS S. Functional and phenotypic plasticity of CD4 (+) T cell subsets [J]. Biomed Res Int, 2015: 521957.

[6] LIU Z, FAN H, JIANG S. CD4 (+) T-cell subsets in transplantation [J]. Immunol Rev, 2013, 252 (1): 183 – 191.

[7] GEGINAT J, PARONI M, MAGLIE S, et al. Plasticity of human CD4 T cell subsets [J]. Front Immunol, 2014, 5: 630.

[8] GEGINAT J, PARONI M, FACCIOTTI F, et al. The CD4-centered universe of human T cell subsets [J]. Semin Immunol, 2013, 25 (4): 252 – 262.

[9] TELLIER J, NUTT SL. The unique features of follicular T cell subsets [J]. Cell Mol Life Sci, 2013, 70 (24): 4771 – 4784.

[10] BERMESTER G R, PEZZUTTO A. Color Atlas of Immunology [M]. New York: Thieme Medical Publishers Inc. , 2003.

[11] SUN B. T helper cell differentiation and their function [M]. Dordrecht: Springer, 2014.

[12] KANEKOS. In vitro differentiation of T cells: methods and protocols [M]. New York: Humana, 2019.

[13] 曹雪涛. 免疫学前沿进展 [M]. 4 版. 北京: 人民卫生出版社, 2017.

[14] 周光炎. 免疫学原理 [M]. 4 版. 北京: 科学出版社, 2018.

[15] BANDO JK, COLONNA M. Innate lymphoid cell function in the context of adaptive immunity [J]. Nat Immunol, 2016, 17 (7): 783 – 789.

（蔡 蓓）

CHAPTER 10
THE HUMORAL IMMUNE RESPONSE AND AUTOIMMUNITY

1 *Words and phrases*

Acquired immune deficiency syndrome（AIDS）　获得性免疫缺陷综合征

Activation　激活

Active immunotherapy　主动免疫治疗

Acute phase protein　急性时相蛋白

Adaptive immunity　适应性免疫（获得性免疫）

Adoptive immunity　过继免疫

Affinity　亲和力

Agglutination　凝集反应

Allergen　变应原

Allergin　变应素

Allergy　变态反应

Allogenic antigen　同种异型抗原

Allograft　同种异型移植，同种异型移植物

Allorecognition　同种异型识别

Allotype　同种异型

Alternative pathway　旁路途径

Ankylosing spondylitis（AS）　强直性脊柱炎

Antibody（Ab）　抗体

Antibody-dependent cell-mediated cytotoxicity（ADCC）
抗体依赖性细胞介导的细胞毒作用

Antigen（Ag）　抗原

Antigen specific immune response　抗原特异性免疫应答

Antigenic determinant　抗原决定簇

Antigen-presenting cell（APC）　抗原提呈细胞

Anti-idiotype　抗独特型

Antinuclear antibodies（ANA） 抗核抗体

Antiphospholipid antibodies 抗磷脂抗体

Antitoxic serum 抗毒素血清

Apoptosis 凋亡

Artificial active immunization 人工主动免疫

Artificial passive immunization 人工被动免疫

Atypical 非典型的

Autoantibodies 自身抗体

Autoimmune diseases 自身免疫病

Autoimmune hemolytic anemia（AIHA） 自身免疫性溶血性贫血

Autoreactive 自身反应

B cell receptor（BCR） B 细胞受体

Lymphocyte 淋巴细胞

Blocking antibody 封闭抗体

Bone marrow 骨髓

Circulating immune complexes（CIC） 循环免疫复合物

Classical pathway 经典途径

Clonal deletion 克隆删除，克隆清除

Co-stimulating signal 共刺激信号

Co-stimulatory molecules 共刺激分子

Cross reaction 交叉反应

Cytokine（CK） 细胞因子

Dendritic cell（DC） 树突状细胞

Disorders 疾病

Double immunodiffusion 双向免疫扩散

Electrophoresis 电泳

Enzyme immunoassay（EIA） 酶免疫分析/试验

Enzyme linked-immunosorbent assay（ELISA） 酶联免疫吸附试验

Erythropoietin（EPO） 促红细胞生成素

Fragment antigen binding（Fab） 抗原结合片段

Germinal center 生发中心

Growth factor 生长因子

Hapten 半抗原

Hashimoto's thyroiditis 桥本甲状腺炎

Heat shock protein（HSP） 热休克蛋白

Heavy chain 重链

Light chain 轻链

Helper T cell 辅助性 T 细胞

Human leukocyte antigen（HLA）　人类白细胞抗原

Humoral immunity　体液免疫

Cellular immunity　细胞免疫

Hypersensitivity　超敏感性

Immunofluorescence　免疫荧光

Indirect immunofluorescence　间接免疫荧光

Immunoglobulin super family　免疫球蛋白超家族

Immunoglobulin（Ig）　免疫球蛋白

Immunohistochemistry technique　免疫组化技术

Immunological tolerance　免疫耐受

Immunology　免疫学

Inflammatory cell　炎症细胞

Innate immunity　固有免疫（天然免疫）

Interferon（IFN）　干扰素

Interleukin（IL）　白介素

Ligand　配体

Lupus nephritis（LN）　狼疮性肾炎

Lymphocyte homing　淋巴细胞归巢

Lymphocyte homing receptor（LHR）　淋巴细胞归巢受体

Membrane attack complex（MAC）　膜攻击复合物

Molecular mimicry　分子模拟

Monoclonal antibody（mcAb）　单克隆抗体

Monocyte　单核细胞

Multiple sclerosis（MS）　多发性硬化症

Myasthenia gravis（MG）　重症肌无力

Natural killer cell（NK cell）　自然杀伤细胞

Organ-specific　器官特异的

Non-organ specific autoimmune disease　非器官特异性自身免疫病

Pathogen　病原体

Plasma cell　浆细胞

Radio immunoassay（RIA）　放射免疫分析

Rejection　排斥

Rheumatoid arthritis（RA）　类风湿关节炎

Rheumatoid factor（RF）　类风湿因子

Secondary immunodeficiency disease（SIDD）　继发性免疫缺陷病

Secondary response　再次应答

Selectin　选择素

Signal transducer and activator of transcription（STAT）　信号转导和活化转录因子

Signal transduction　信号转导

Single immunodiffusion　单向免疫扩散

Super antigen　超抗原

Systemic lupus erythematosus　系统性红斑狼疮

Tumor necrosis factor（TNF）　肿瘤坏死因子

Vaccine　疫苗

Western blotting　免疫印迹法

2　*Readings*

2.1　Introduction

Humoral immunity is of great importance in both healthy people and patients. It is critical that vaccine stimulates antibodies and mediates protection against pathogens in host defense.

　　Antibodies, which are considered as production in response to antigens, play key roles in fighting infection. Immunoglobulins (Ig) are originally demonstrated by serum electrophoresis to reside in the gamma globulin fraction of human serum. The basic structure of the antibody consists of 2 light and 2 heavy glycoprotein chains which are joined together by an interchain. There are 5 types of heavy chains, including gamma (IgG), mu (IgM), alpha (IgA), delta (IgD), and epsilon (IgE), and 2 types of light chains including kappa and lambda. In general, IgG has the highest concentration in serum, but IgM, IgA, IgD, and IgE with lighter concentrations respectively.

　　Normally, the immune system "tolerates" to the self-tissues of the host. However, the immune system appears abnormal under pathological conditions, such as systemic lupus erythematosus (SLE), rheumatoid arthritis (RA), myasthenia gravis (MG), multiple sclerosis (MS), and autoimmune hemolytic anemia (AIHA). Till now there are over 40 diseases considered to be autoimmune diseases in nature, affecting about 5% population in the world. Autoimmune diseases predominate in females. The risk of some autoimmune diseases may be increased eight times in women. However, there are notable exceptions such as ankylosing spondylitis (AS). Autoimmune diseases also show genetic evidence of clustering within families.

　　As chronic illnesses, interactions between genetic and environmental factors are very important in the causation of autoimmune diseases. Family studies have confirmed genetic contribution in autoimmune diseases. Multiple autoimmune diseases patients may cluster in the same family and genetic contribution to autoimmune diseases always involves many genes. Some genes involve defects in apoptosis or clearing of circulating immune complexes (CIC). Environmental factors are identified as possible triggers in autoimmunity including hormones, infections, drugs, and ultraviolet radiations.

Hormones, as one of the most striking epidemiological observations regarding autoimmune diseases , are far more affected in females than males. Most autoimmune diseases have their peak age of onset within the reproductive years. The study evidence suggests that oestrogens can stimulate certain types of the immune responses. The pituitary hormone prolactin also has immunostimulatory actions, particularly on T cells.

In addition, infection is the clearest factor in the pathogenesis of autoimmune diseases through molecular mimicry. Infection of target organ may play a key role in local up-regulation of co-stimulatory molecules and also in inducing altered patterns of antigen breakdown and presentation, thus leading to autoimmunity without molecular mimicry.

The autoimmune pathological process may be initiated by autoantibodies, immune complexes (IC) containing autoantigens, and autoreactive T lymphocytes. Each of them plays a preponderant role in certain diseases. Sometimes they may be synergistically associated and cause multiorgan autoimmune diseases. B lymphocytes with autoreactive specificities remain non-deleted in adult individuals and lead to the production of autoantibodies such as antinuclear antibodies (ANA). In general, it is polyclonal B-cell activation that may be associated with the activation of autoreactive B lymphocytes. Autoantibody-associated diseases are characterized by the deposition of autoantibodies in tissues. Autoantibodies may be directly involved in the pathogenesis of some diseases, while in others, they may serve simply as disease markers, without a known pathogenic role. For example, the anti-Sm antibody found unique in SLE patients is unclear of pathogenic role.

Autoimmune diseases can affect any organ in the body. Conventionally autoimmune diseases have been classified into organ-specific and non-organ-specific disorders. Usually, organ-specific autoimmune disorders affect one organ and the autoimmune response is directed against multiple antigens located in the organ. Non-organ-specific autoimmune diseases affect multiple organs and autoimmune responses against self-molecules are widely distributed through the body. Many of these non-organ-specific disorders are labeled as " connective tissue diseases"; this is a misleading term since the " connective tissues" is neither abnormal nor specifically damaged, but the term is used widely.

Autoantibodies are antibodies against tissues, organs, cells, and cellular components. There are many autoantibodies in autoimmune diseases, of which the most important is ANA. ANA is a group of many kinds of autoantibodies. ANA detection is important to the evaluation of patients with a broad range of autoimmune diseases. ANA target components such as dsDNA, RNA, and proteins, etc. The number of ANA specificities is large and some antibodies are highly related to particular diseases, but most are expressed widely among patients. The high association between ANA and certain disease suggests that these antibodies could be used as good biomarkers for screening and diagnosis of disease, and it also could provide insights for understanding disease mechanisms. ANA testing has been used as a central test in rheumatology for over 50 years, but many aspects of these popular biomarkers remain a matter of uncertainty and even controversy. ANA positivity was initially seen as notable in the criterion of SLE. At present, ANA positivity occurs so commonly in patients with musculoskeletal complaints and vague symptomatology. One positive result might be neither revealing nor informative.

ANA, as autoantibodies, can bind to nuclear antigens sharing a similar sequence or structure from different species. ANA can be divided into two groups. One group consists of antibodies that recognize DNA, histones, and nucleosomes. The other can bind to complexes of RNA with RNA-binding proteins (RBPs). Examples of ANA recognizing RBPs include anti-Sm, anti-RNP, anti-Ro, and anti-La antibodies. Anti-Ro60 binds to the protein component of a complex comprising small cytoplasmic RNA molecules; by contrast, anti-Ro52 recognizes a member of the tripartite motif (TRIM) family, which is a ubiquitin ligase not forming RNA or protein complexes. Although most of the nuclear antigens targeted by ANA are present in the cell nucleus, these molecules are mobile and can translocate to the cytoplasm even to the extracellular space. These translocations most prominently occur during apoptosis. In the extracellular space, nuclear antigens can form immune complexes with ANA which can stimulate immune responses, such as the production of type I interferon. In other words, immune complexes can exert important pathogenic activities. Therefore, to some extent, ANA testing, especially for antibodies of certain specificities (such as anti-DNA and anti-RBP antibodies), can provide valuable information on pathogenic pathways that might be involved in various autoimmune diseases.

Although the ANA test is useful to assess the likelihood of a diagnosis of autoimmune disease, much more useful information comes from the identification of the target antigens bound by ANA, with certain antibodies strongly associated with particular diseases. Important associations include anti-dsDNA and anti-Sm antibodies with SLE; anti-topoisomerase I antibodies with progressive systemic sclerosis; anti-Jo-1 antibodies with myositis and anti-centromere antibodies with a limited cutaneous form of systemic sclerosis. In contrast to the disease specificity of some ANA, anti-Ro60, and anti-Ro52 commonly occur in SLE and rheumatoid arthritis (RA), despite being an important feature of Sjögren syndrome. Nevertheless, positivity to anti-RNP antibodies is not considered a classification criterion for SLE diagnosis because these antibodies are also found in mixed connective tissue disease (MCTD). The anti-RNP antibodies are considered important in the diagnosis of MCTD. In the clinic, the patient who is positive for ANA, the presence of a specific ANA increases the likelihood of a diagnosis of disease depending on the clinical and laboratory findings. Now ANA has been detected by immunofluorescence assay (IFA) recommended for about 50 years as an important application of fluorescent antibody technology. IFA is simple in principle, and involves incubation of serum or plasma samples with a source of cells, either a tissue section or a cell line fixed to a glass slide. At present, the HEp-2 cell is used widely due to a variety of antigens. In IFA, the presence of antibodies is assessed by a fluoresceinated anti-IgG reagent. In general, the frequency of ANA positivity of SLE patients is considered up to 95% − 99%.

The patterns of fluorescence observed in IFA might also provide insight into the specificity of ANA of target antigens. In this regard, given that entire cells are used for antibody detection, antibodies to nuclear molecules, mitotic and cytoplasmic can also be detected simultaneously. Common patterns detected by IFA include speckled, homogeneous, nucleolar, and rim patterns. In past, IFA is often regarded as the "gold standard" for serological ANA test. Unfortunately, the performance of IFA can indeed be subject to variability related to the assay kit used, conditions of cell fixation, cellular concentration, the specificity of the anti-IgG, and starting dilution of sera used for testing. By its nature, IFA is a visual test and depends upon the observer. Especially for sera with low titers of antibodies, the assignment of positivity might differ among different observers. Of note, the amounts of certain autoantigens in HEp-2 cells, such as Ro60, can limit the detection of antibodies against this molecule. A modified cell line HEp-2000 transfected with Ro60 complementary DNA and expressing more Ro60 protein can detect of anti-Ro60 antibodies more sensitivity than HEp-2 cell. Studies have demonstrated that ANA negativity occurs frequently in SLE. The number of SLE patients who are negative for ANA can range from 5% to 20%, one reason is depending on the assay kit used differently.

Enzyme linked-immunosorbent assay (ELISA) is one of the most popular and versatile analytical techniques in the validation of ANA detection through mixed or crude antigens. The advantages of this approach include easy utilization, the possibility to perform quantitative and high-throughput analyses. The main disadvantages related to uncertainty in the content of certain antigens and a lack of information on the specificity of antibodies. Although IFA does not provide precise information about the specificity of antibodies in serum, it can indicate the identity of antibodies through the binding pattern. ELISA can also be used to detect specific ANA such as anti-Ro and anti-La antibodies, etc.

Recently several multiplex assays are available for the simultaneous detection of ANA recognizing nuclear autoantigens. Among these assays, line immunoassay is a useful technique for detecting antibodies to specific autoantigens. In line immunoassay, a limited selection of antigens including purified proteins, recombinant proteins, or synthetic peptides are coated in parallel lines to a nylon membrane strip. The nylon membrane is incubated with diluted sera from patients, antibodies are detected by an anti-IgG reagent conjugated to an enzyme. In addition, multiplex assay with addressable beads is a more recent and technologically sophisticated approach to detect antibodies. It utilizes a series of beads of distinct immunofluorescence intensities and is coated with different purified antigens. The antibodies against different antigens can be determined by flow cytometry. If the test shows positivity for antibodies to any antigen, the serum is considered to be "screen positive". Similar to the line immunoassay, the multiplex bead-based assay assesses the binding of only a limited subset of ANA, therefore, it will miss many of the less-common specific types of autoantibodies from patients with myositis. Other technologies such as chip-based assay can provide serological assessments in greater detail. These assays can measure hundreds of antibodies. The broad analysis of autoantibody binding provided by chip-based assay provides more autoreactivity results than before and provides more possibilities for screening autoantibodies.

Now ANA test is one of the most important tests because a positive result represents a high possibility for the diagnosis of autoimmune disease, while ANA positivity is present in a substantial proportion of the healthy population. By contrast, assays directed to particular autoantigens such as dsDNA provide more specific biomarkers. Despite its shortcomings, the ANA test will remain commonly performed to evaluate patients with musculoskeletal complaints. Future assays that utilize a larger panel of autoantigens may provide useful information in clinic.

2. 2　Systemic lupus erythematosus

Systemic lupus erythematosus (SLE) is a multisystem disorder affecting young women frequently. It is characterized by the presence of ANA. The most common presenting symptom is arthritis or arthralgia. Nearly all patients eventually experience joint problems and skin lesions while some have pulmonary, renal, neurological, and hematological involvement. New pieces of evidence have been found on the relationship between genetic polymorphisms and environment in contribution to SLE pathogenesis in Chinese. The result showed that the polymorphism rs2234693 of Estrogen Receptor alpha gene (*ESR1*) increased the risk of SLE in smoking patients compared to non-smokers. To investigate the clinical value of anti-Sm antibodies in diagnosis and monitoring of SLE, although no correlations with lupus activity were observed in the longitudinal and predictive analysis, a remarkable association was found between anti-Sm and proteinuria, suggesting that anti-Sm monitoring was helpful in SLE patients with active lupus nephritis (LN). Recently a prospective longitudinal benchmark study revealed that IFN-γ-inducible protein-10 (IP-10) could be considered as an excellent biomarker for monitoring disease activity. The serum levels significantly increased during flares and decreased during remissions. This is an important finding because other traditional biomarkers do not have such versatility in reflecting longitudinal changes in disease activity.

Atypical SLE often causes difficulty in diagnosis. Pericarditis is the commonest cardiac lesion and is usually transient and mild. A heart murmur can be due to the classical endocarditis of SLE. Anaemia, fever, and tachycardia are more frequent causes. Similarly, pleurisy and pneumonitis are common but mild and transient. The renal complications and neurological features of SLE have been increasingly recognized, particularly with the advent of nuclear magnetic resonance imaging. The prognosis in SLE has improved dramatically over the last 25 years. For all forms of SLE, the 5-year survival figure exceeds 90%. Even in patients with proven nephritis, the 5-year survival is now over 80%. Pregnancy is not contraindicated, although spontaneous abortion and stillbirths are more frequent, an additional congenital heart block hazard to the fetus is associated with maternal antibodies to Ro. About laboratory tests, SLE patients have ANA, including antibodies to dsDNA. A negative ANA does not exclude a suspected diagnosis of SLE, while positive dsDNA antibodies strongly support it. Because of the wide range of presenting symptoms and the difficulties of making a definite diagnosis, all patients in whom SLE are suspected should be tested for ANA, including anti-dsDNA, anti-Sm, anti-rib, and antiphospholipid antibodies, as well as detect their serum levels of Ig and complement components (C3 and C4).

Due to the increasing complexity of ANA testing, groups such as the Autoantibody Standardization Committee, a subcommittee of the Quality Assessment and Standardization Committee of the International Union of Immunological Societies (IUIS), have been established to address the importance of standardization in ANA test. It is helpful in diagnosis and differential diagnosis in autoimmune disease. (Figure 10 − 1)

Corticosteroids plus cytotoxic agents have been the standard of care for the treatment of SLE for decades. For the first 3 − 5 years after treatment initiation, the study showed that corticosteroids and cyclophosphamide were equally effective. Due to concerns related to cyclophosphamide toxicity, it was designed using low-dose, substituting mycophenolate mofetil (MMF) for cyclophosphamide, or combining a calcineurin inhibitor with MMF and corticosteroids. Low-dose cyclophosphamide and MMF were found to be equivalent to standard cyclophosphamide, whereas multitarget therapy with cyclosporine, MMF, and corticosteroids appeared to be superior to cyclophosphamide for short-term remission induction.

To date, belimumab (anti-BLyS) is the FDA-approved biologic for treating. Currently, drugs representing a variety of therapeutic strategies are moving to phase Ⅲ trials. These include cytokine infusions (low dose IL-2); antibodies against cytokines (ustekinumab); and finally, small molecule inhibitors against kinases (Jak inhibitors) and phosphatases (calcineurin inhibitors). Combinatorial therapies targeting offer the potential of abrogating inflammation to improve short-term response rates and prevent disease recurrence and progressive kidney failure.

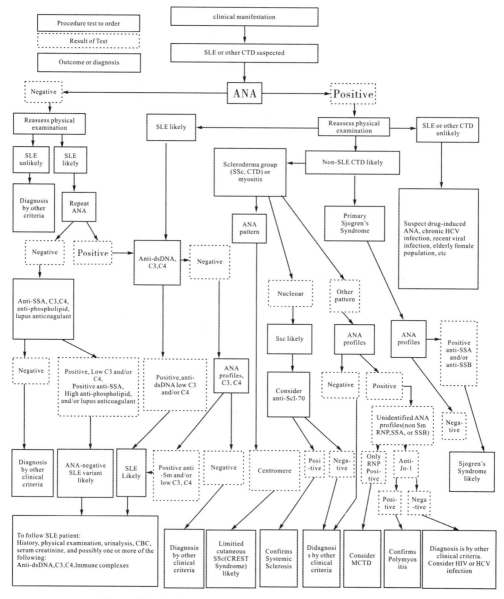

Figure 10 - 1　Laboratory diagnosis of autoimmune diseases.

3　Discussion

A 26-year-old woman presented with painful, stiff knees of 4 weeks' duration. She had a 6-year history of Raynaud's phenomenon. On examination, she had bilateral effusions in both knee joints, and other joints were normal. She had no skin lesions, muscle tenderness, proteinuria or fever. Antinuclear antibody was positive at 1/320, C3 and C4 levels were occasionally low.

(1) What diseases might the patient have?

(2) What further tests should be done?

References and resources

[1] EWART D, PETERSON EJ, STEER CJ. A new era of genetic engineering for autoimmune and inflammatorydiseases [J]. Semin Arthritis Rheum. 2019: 49 (1): e1 - e7.

[2] KHODADADI L, CHENG Q, RADBRUCH A, et al. The maintenance of memory plasma cells [J]. Front Immunol, 2019, 5 (10): 721.

[3] WU Y, VAN BESOUW NM, SHI Y, et al. The biological effects of IL-21 signaling on B-cell-mediated responses in organ transplantation [J]. Front Immunol, 2016, 23 (7): 319.

[4] WU Y, CAI B, ZHANG J, et al. IL-1β and IL-6 are highly expressed in RF + IgE + systemic lupus erythematous subtype [J]. J Immunol Res, 2017: 5096741.

[5] MENG Y, DENG S, HUANG Z, et al. Evaluating the diagnostic and prognostic value of lone anti-Sm for autoimmune diseases using Euroimmun line immunoassays [J]. Clin Rheumatol, 2018 , 37 (11): 3017 - 3023.

[6] DSOUZA L, BHATTACHARYA D. Plasma cells: you are what you eat [J]. Immunol Rev, 2019, 288 (1): 161 - 177.

[7] LEIBLER C, THIOLAT A, ELSNER R A, et al. Costimulatory blockade molecules and B-cell-mediated immune response: current knowledge and perspectives [J]. Kidney Int, 2019 , 95 (4): 774 - 786.

[8] STEBEGG M, KUMAR S D, SILVA-CAYETANO A, et al. Regulation of the germinal center response [J]. Front Immunol, 2018, 9: 2469.

[9] DOHERTY D G, MELO A M, MORENO-OLIVERA A, et al. Activation and regulation of B cell responses by invariant natural killer T cells [J]. Front Immunol, 2018 , 9: 1360.

[10] WU Y, HOOGDUIJN M J, BAAN C C, et al. Adipose tissue-derived mesenchymal stem cells have a heterogenic cytokine secretion profile [J]. Stem Cells Int, 2017: 4960831.

[11] MENG Y, XU H, ZHANG S, et al. Genetic polymorphisms near IL-21 gene associated with Th17 cytokines confer risk for systemic lupus erythematosus in Chinese Han population [J]. Lupus. 2019, 28 (3): 406 - 413.

[12] PISETSKY D S. Antinuclear antibody testing-misunderstood or misbegotten? [J]. Nat Rev Rheumatol, 2017, 13 (8): 495 - 502.

[13] DI BATTISTA M, MARCUCCI E, ELEFANTE E, et al. One year in review 2018: systemic lupus erythematosus [J]. Clin Exp Rheumatol, 2018, 36 (5): 763 - 777.

[14] JELLUSOVA J. Metabolic control of B cell immune responses [J]. Curr Opin

Immunol, 2020, 63: 21 - 28.

[15] FINNEY J, WATANABE A, KELSOE G, et al. Minding the gap: the impact of B-cell tolerance on the microbial antibody repertoire [J]. Immunol Rev, 2019, 292 (1): 24 - 36.

[16] TAYLOR H, LAURENCE A D J, UHLIG H H. The Role of PTEN in innate and adaptive immunity [J]. Cold Spring Harb Perspect Med, 2019, 9 (12): a036996.

[17] KIM J H, KIM S C. Paraneoplastic pemphigus: paraneoplastic autoimmune disease of the skin and mucosa [J]. Front Immunol, 2019, 4; 10: 1259.

[18] MENG Y, HE Y, ZHANG J, et al. Association of GTF2I gene polymorphisms with renal involvement of systemic lupus erythematosus in a Chinese population [J]. Medicine (Baltimore), 2019, 98 (31): e16716.

[19] BEN MKADDEM S, BENHAMOU M, MONTEIRO R C. Understanding Fc receptor involvement in inflammatory diseases: from mechanisms to new therapeutic tools [J]. Front Immunol, 2019, 10: 811.

[20] ISE W, KUROSAKI T. Plasma cell differentiation during the germinal center reaction [J]. Immunol Rev, 2019, 288 (1): 64 - 74.

[21] MYLES A, SANZ I, CANCRO MP. T-bet (+) B cells: a common denominator in protective and autoreactive antibody responses? [J] Curr Opin Immunol, 2019, 57: 40 - 45.

[22] LEIBLER C, THIOLAT A, ELSNER R A, et al. Costimulatory blockade molecules and B-cell-mediated immune response: current knowledge and perspectives [J]. Kidney Int, 2019, 95 (4): 774 - 786.

[23] KARNELL J L, RIEDER S A, ETTINGER R, et al. Targeting the CD40 - CD40L pathway in autoimmune diseases: humoral immunity and beyond [J]. Adv Drug Deliv Rev, 2019, 141: 92 - 103.

[24] WANG S, MENG Y, HUANG Z, et al. Anti-centrosome antibodies: prevalence and disease association in Chinese population [J]. Scand J Immunol, 2019, 90 (4): e12803.

（武永康）

CHAPTER 11
LABORATORY DIAGNOSIS OF INFECTIOUS DISEASES

1　*Words and phrases*

Bacteria　细菌

Fungus　真菌

Yeast　酵母菌

Virus　病毒

Mycoplasma　支原体

Chlamydia　衣原体

Parasite　寄生虫

Microbiology　微生物学

Bacteriology　细菌学

Virology　病毒学

Mycology　真菌学

Parasitology　寄生虫学

Serology　血清学

Microscopic examination　显微镜检查

Smear　涂片

Gram stain　革兰染色

Media　培养基

Aerobe　需氧菌

Anaerobe　厌氧菌

Isolation　分离

Culture　培养

Species identification　菌种鉴定

Genus　属

Species　种

Strain　株

Antimicrobial susceptibility testing（AST）　抗微生物药物敏感试验

Antimicrobial agents　抗微生物制剂

Diffusion　稀释法

Agar　琼脂

Broth　肉汤

Resistant（R）　耐药的

Intermediate（I）　中介的

Susceptible（S）　敏感的

susceptible-dose dependent（SDD）　剂量依赖性敏感的

Matrix-assisted laser desorption/Ionization time-of-flight mass spectrometry（MALDI－TOF MS）　基质辅助激光解吸电离飞行时间质谱

Phenotype　表型

Genotype　基因型

Sequencing　测序

Disinfection　消毒

Sterilization　灭菌

Antiseptic　防腐剂

Microbiome　微生物组

Pathogen　病原体

Etiology　病原学

Flora　菌群

Colonization　定植

Infection　感染

Nosocomial infection　院内感染

Hospital-acquired　医院获得的

Community-acquired　社区获得的

Bloodstream infection　血流感染

Urinary tract infection　尿路感染

Respiratory tract infection　呼吸道感染

Bacteremia　菌血症

Toxemia　毒血症

Pneumonia　肺炎

Endocarditis　心内膜炎

Meningitis　脑膜炎

2   *Readings*

2.1   Introduction

2.1.1   Infectious diseases

Global health has been steadily improved over the past several decades. While, the infectious diseases, caused by the organisms (bacteria, viruses, fungi, parasites, etc.), remain a heavy burden for mankind. For example, acquired immune deficiency syndrome (AIDS), hepatitis C, and tuberculosis (TB) are killing millions of people each year. Increasing antimicrobial resistance has become a big challenge for the management of infectious diseases. Multidrug resistant organisms (MDROs), such as carbapenem-resistant *Enterobacteriaceae* (CRE), methicillin-resistant *Staphylococcus aureus* (MRSA), and vancomycin-resistant *Enterococcus* (VRE), have become the emergent threat announced by World Health Organization (WHO). Furthermore, some diseases, like those caused by the Ebola virus, multidrug-resistant tuberculosis (MDR-TB), avian/swine influenza, severe acute respiratory syndrome (SARS), Middle East respiratory syndrome (MERS), and coronavirus disease 2019 (COVID - 19), have brought major public health consequences.

There are some challenges for the physicians to diagnosis the patients suspected of infectious diseases. Firstly, the same pathogen is often capable of causing a variety of clinical manifestations. Secondly, some clinical syndromes can be caused by many and quite different pathogens. Lastly, some infectious diseases can resemble the non-infectious diseases. Therefore, the detection of the samples from the patients in the clinical laboratories are critically important for the diagnosis of infectious diseases. Several indicators, such as count and classification of white blood cells, procalcitonin (PCT), interleukin-6 (IL-6), C reaction protein (CRP), are used for assisting their diagnosis. Microbiological detection of the samples is performed to provide the etiological basis.

2.1.2   Clinical microbiology

Clinical microbiology has been established since Hooke invented the microscope in 1665, and then was facilitated by some milestones. For example, Pasteur discovered the presence of pathogenic organisms in infected patients. Koch established three principles to determine the causal relationship between organisms and diseases. Gram invented Gram staining to benefit the detection of the organisms through a light microscope. Perry devised a petri dish to culture some kind of organisms in vitro.

At present, clinical microbiology has become a discipline that can determine whether the presence of pathogens in patient's samples or not and provide antimicrobial resistance profiles of the isolated organisms. Also, it provides consulting services, including interpreting report involving in epidemiological investigation of an infection outbreak, and participating in antimicrobial stewardship.

In clinical laboratories, both the traditional and newly-developed techniques have been applied to analyze the patients' samples, and the detection results are referred to the management of infectious diseases.

2.1.3 Microbiological techniques

1. Microscopic examination

Microscopic examination is performed to rapidly screen the potential pathogens in specimens. The direct microscopy, microscopy after staining (e.g. Gram staining, India ink staining, and fluorescent staining), electron microscopy, etc., can be used according to the species suspected. For example, Gram-negative diplococci inner and external leukocyte cell observed in the smearing of male genital tract secretion suggest the presence of *Neisseria gonorrhea* (Figure 11 – 1). Circled bacterial cells around with transparent and thick capsules in cerebrospinal fluid specimens stained with India ink, indicate the existence of *Cryptococcus* species (Figure 11 – 2). Whereas, low sensitivity is the major disadvantage for microscopic examination technique.

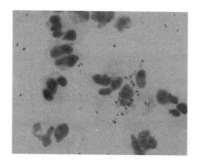

Figure 11 – 1 *Neisseria gonorrhea* **stained with Gram dye** (×1000). (see Appendix Figure 16)

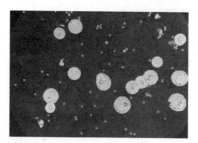

Figure 11 – 2 *Cryptococcus* **spp. stained with India ink** (×1000). (see Appendix Figure 17)

2. Isolation and culture

Isolation and culture of the pathogens from patients' samples are regarded as the "gold standard" techniques for the etiological diagnosis of infectious diseases. At first, inanimate media for extracellular organisms (e. g. bacteria, fungi, Figure 11 − 3), or living media for intracellular ones (e. g. virus, chlamydia), are applied to isolate the organisms from the specimens. Ideally, the culture should be performed before antimicrobial agents are administered. Samples should be collected appropriately according to the location and type of the infection suspected and sent to the laboratories as soon as possible. The operation process of isolation and culture technique can vary dramatically, depending on the organism that is being sought.

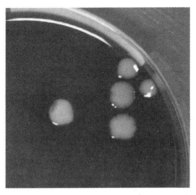

(a) *Staphylococcus aureus* on the blood agar plate. (35℃, 2 days)

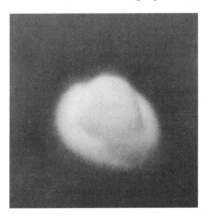

(b) *Beauveria* spp. on the potato-dextrose plate. (28℃, 7 days)

Figure 11 − 3   Colony morphorogy of some organisms on inanimate media (see Appendix Figure 18)

3. Species identification

Traditionally, a battery of biochemical reactions can be performed for the species identification of bacterial strains. For instance, members of *Enterobacteriales* can be identified by a battery of 14 tests, including gas from glucose, indole production, lysine decarboxylase, motility, adonitol fermentation, arginine dihydrolase, citrate utilization, sucrose fermentation, urease, DNAase, hydrogen sulfide, ornithine decarboxylase, phenylalanine deaminase, and Voges-

Proskauer. This kind of battery test is sufficient for the identification of the most clinically significant *Enterobacteriales* to the genus level and of many isolates to the species level. Currently, these tests can be integrated into commercial kits and incubated in automated identification systems for improving their applicability. Generally, biochemical reactions require about hours to days to achieve results and are not suitable for fastidious organisms.

A novel technique, matrix-assisted laser desorption/ionization time-of-flight mass spectrometry (MALDI-TOF MS), has been adapted for microbial identification. It involves using a laser to vaporize and ionize molecules, measuring the molecules' mass-to-charge ratios (m/z), and generating a mass spectrum using time-of-flight mass spectrometry. The organisms are analyzed with or without a preceding extraction step. A characteristic mass spectrum of the unknown strain is produced and compared to the reference database with mass spectra generated from known organisms. The unknown strain is identified to the genus or species level based on the closest match. This kind of technique is allowing accurate identification of a large variety of bacterial species within a few minutes and with only a small amount of culture sample required for the analysis ($10^4 - 10^6$ CFU). Furthermore, it is easy to use, and has high accuracy. However, it must be noted that the results are limited by the reference databases, which require regular updating.

Additionally, amplifying and sequencing of specific genetic elements [e. g. 16s RNA for bacterial strains, internal transcribed spacer (ITS) for fungal strains], or whole-genome sequencing can be applied for identifying the isolated organisms.

4. Antimicrobial susceptibility testing

For the identified strain, antimicrobial susceptibility testing (AST) is performed to assess whether it is susceptible to antimicrobial agents or not. In practice, phenotypic testing, including disk diffusion, broth microdilution, and gradient diffusion, are conventionally used and the results are interpreted as susceptible (S), intermediate (I), susceptible-dose dependent (SDD), or resistant (R), if the operation procedures and breakpoints for the species are available in the standardized documents.

In addition, MALDI-TOF MS come to be used to analyze antimicrobial resistance. Genetic mutations associated with resistance can be identified by genotypic assays, which have almost completely replaced phenotypic testing for viral pathogens. Importantly, clinical laboratories must give high priority not only to producing accurate data but also to reporting those data to physicians in an interpretable manner for guiding treatment options.

5. Immunoassay

Immunoassays, examining specific antigens of some organisms and the body response against them, are often conducted for early-stage screening or epidemiological investigation, but the results are typically not used as the sole basis on which a diagnosis is made.

Whereas, for certain diseases, such as cryptococcal meningitis, Lyme disease, and syphilis, antibody or antigen detection is the primary technique by which the infection is established. Due to ease of use, short turnaround time and generally high specificity, these assays are extensively developed as point-of-care testings (POCTs).

6. Nucleotide acid detection

The sensitivity and specificity of nucleotide acid-based techniques, such as polymerase chain reaction (PCR), nucleic acid hybridization, sequencing, are higher than those of microbial culture. Moreover, these kinds of culture-independent techniques are especially suitable for the detection of culture-difficult organisms in the specimens. Currently, these techniques have been extensively used in clinical practice.

For instance, multiplex PCR, enabling the simultaneous detection of multiple pathogens without additional time or sampling, can be used to rapidly screen the common pathogens associated with certain body systems, such as blood stream, respiratory tract, and urinary tract.

Microbial genomic sequencing can be applied to yield a comprehensive understanding of the genetic characteristics of the pathogens, including their evolution and key genes for virulence and resistance.

Metagenomic next-generation sequencing (mNGS) includes multiple steps, namely sample collection, nucleic acid extraction, library construction, sequencing, and bioinformatics analysis. It is promising for rapid screening of numerous organisms in specimens and especially useful for identifying rare species, which are helpful for the diagnosis of complicated infections. Such applications have already begun and are expected to grow. Whereas, high cost, complicated operation, probable contamination, and difficult results interpretation are the challenges.

7. Conclusion

Traditional microbiological techniques that relied substantially on culture have been supplanted in part by novel methods including protein analysis, nucleic acid detection and specific molecular test.

POCT platforms have been developed for rapid screening of the pathogens. However, further optimization and clinical verifications are required to enhance their performance for the detection of clinical specimens.

In this era of metagenomics medicine, the ability of high-throughput nucleic acid-based techniques to rapidly screen microbial genetic materials will continue to bring a profound impact on our understanding of the pathogenesis of infectious diseases. The findings will promote the development of diagnostic techniques for infectious diseases.

2. 2　Laboratory diagnosis of lower respiratory tract infections (LRTIs)

2. 2. 1　Overview

Low respiratory tract infections (LRTIs), including bronchitis, bronchiolitis, pneumonia, and pleural infections, are the most common infectious diseases. In 2019, World Health Organization declared that LRTIs and tuberculosis were the top 4 and 9 cause of global deaths respectively. In this chapter, we will focus on the microbiological approach to LRTIs diagnosis, but that of tuberculosis will be described in chapter 12 of this book.

LRTIs can be caused by viruses, bacteria, fungi, mycoplasmas, etc. Traditionally, physicians formulate a differential diagnosis of the diseases from a constellation of clinical signs and symptoms, while LRTIs are usually indistinguishable based on clinical features alone. Also, the etiology of LRTIs is significantly different across different countries, regions, populations, and changes over time. So, diagnostic tests are necessary for guiding precise treatment of the patients suspected of LRTIs.

For accurate pathogen identification, collecting appropriate samples from the patients is the first step. Respiratory tract samples [e. g. nasopharyngeal swab, sputum, tracheal aspirate, bronchoalveolar lavage fluid (BALF)], pleural fluid, tissue, and/or blood samples are commonly collected. Secondly, the selection of diagnostic tests should take into account multiple factors, such as epidemiological features, demographic data, underlying diseases, immune status, clinical characteristics, the severity of disease and prior anti-infective treatment. Last but not least, the results of diagnostic tests should be reviewed comprehensively before being sent to the physicians.

2. 2. 2　Bacterial LRTIs

Microscopic examination, isolation, and culture are the routine microbiological investigations for bacterial causes of LRTIs. The first morning expectorated sputum is a readily available sample. But, the sputum might be contaminated with upper respiratory tract-colonizing organisms. The quality of sputum samples should be assessed before further handling. Qualified sputum samples must meet the following condition in per low power field of microscopy: number of squamous cells is < 10, number of polymorphonuclear leukocytes is > 25; or the ratio of squamous cells to polymorphonuclear leukocytes is $< 1 : 2. 5$. One way to avoid the consequence of such contamination is the use of BALF culture, but this procedure is invasive and therefore limited to specialized units.

Sometimes, blood culture can be used when LRTIs are suspected. Whereas, its role is limited given that infection is generally localized to lung parenchyma and cultures may be taken with concomitant antibiotic use. So, blood culture is suggested for patients with severe LRTIs or in high-risk populations.

In this context, result interpretation of samples for bacterial investigation is challenging. Test results can be used as the evidence for etiological diagnosis in the following settings: (1) The pathogen is found in cultures of blood or other sterile samples (such as pleural effusion, lung biopsy samples); (2) Francisella tularensis, Bacillus anthracis, or Yersinia pestis is isolated from qualified lower respiratory tract samples. Test results are important references for etiological diagnosis in the following settings: (1) Significant growth of dominant bacteria in qualified lower respiratory tract samples (except for normal colonization flora) is observed; (2) Small amount of bacterial clones grow in qualified lower respiratory tract samples, but these results are consistent with smear microscopy results; (3) Apparent bacterial phagocytosis by neutrophils could be seen in smear microscopy of qualified lower respiratory tract samples.

2.2.3   Viral LRTIs

A positive result for viral isolation and culture is the "gold standard" for the diagnosis of viral infection, but this kind of technique is time-consuming and sometimes has low specificity. Also, it requires proper specimen collection and transportation to prevent the loss of viability of the viruses before arrival in laboratory. Therefore, more practical tests are preferred in clinical laboratories.

The common respiratory viruses can be identified by detecting specific viral antigens in nasopharyngeal specimens (swabs, aspirates, or washes). Rapid antigen detection testing (RADT) for these viruses (e.g. influenza virus) can often provide the results in less than 30 minutes, but their sensitivity is only 40% to 70% (specificity is >90%). While RADT is still in conventional use as an initial screening method for early-stage diagnosis due to its low cost and fast results. Epidemiological history and clinical symptoms of the patient should be taken into account when interpreting the results. Nucleic acid detection or viral isolation and culture can be performed for further validation if necessary.

Immunofluorescent assays in which slides are stained with labeled antibodies are much more sensitive. However, they are labor-intensive and require skilled technicians.

Over the past 2 decades, clinical virology diagnosis has been revolutionized with the introduction of nucleic acid-based techniques. Commercially available nucleic acid amplification assays (e.g. real-time PCR, real-time reverse transcriptase PCR) can detect several respiratory viruses in 1 to 8 hours and the rival can exceed the sensitivity and specificity of viral culture. Panel assays were also applied to rapidly screen a series of viruses associated with LRTIs. These techniques have greatly improved the performance of laboratory diagnosis of respiratory viral infection and facilitated the finding that viral pathogens are more frequently associated with LRTIs.

2.2.4   Fungal LRTIs

Microscopic examination, often with Gram staining for yeast or calcofluor white staining for filamentous fungi, is a kind of conventional method for detecting the fungi in respiratory tract samples. Besides, Giemsa staining can be used for the detection of human Pneumocystis. Microscopy with KOH as floating fluid can be used to detect hypha and spores of fungi.

Serum 1-3-β-D glucan antigen test (G test) provides the reference for the diagnosis of invasive fungal infections, except for Cryptococcus and Zygomycetes-associated infections. Serum or BALF galactomannan antigen test (GM test) has important value for the diagnosis of invasive pulmonary aspergillosis.

Isolation and cultivation are commonly requested for respiratory tract samples, but fungal growth is usually not detected for several days to weeks. Morphologic tests and nucleic acid detection are usually performed for the identification of the strains. A positive result for the fungal culture of a sample from a usually sterile site using an aseptic technique can provide the basis of diagnosis. For non-sterile samples, the possibility of colonization or pollution should be carefully excluded.

In practice, the diagnosis of respiratory fungal infections should combine the results of diagnostic tests, clinical presentation, and demonstration of characteristic structures in biopsy specimens.

2.2.5 Atypical pathogens associated LRTIs

For atypical pathogens (e. g. *Mycoplasma* spp. , *Chlamydia* spp. , *Legionella* pneumophila) , a positive result of culture can be used to establish a definite diagnosis of LRTIs, but the test is time-consuming, and the positive rate is relatively low.

Serological testing of specific immunoglobulin M (IgM) or immunoglobulin G (IgG) is used as a routine detection. Serum specific IgM appears in the early stage of the disease, but acute infection could not be excluded by a negative result. A quadruple or higher increase in IgG titer across two sets of serum samples is relevant for retrospective diagnostic.

Nucleic acid assays of these pathogens in respiratory tract samples have been approved for clinical use, and positive results have value for early-stage diagnosis.

2.2.6 Parasites associated LRTIs

If the clinical and epidemiologic data suggest parasites associated LRTIs. Direct microscopic examination of pleural fluid and sputum for characteristic ova or worm, and Giemsa-stained smear of pleural fluid, or biopsy can be performed. Serological assays and molecular-based detection of the samples can be carried out when the related reagents are available. Due to the high requirements and long periods for the cultivation of parasites, these pathogens cannot routinely be isolated and identified in most clinical microbiology laboratories.

2.2.7 Challenge

Though the exciting advances of diagnostic techniques for LRTIs have been made in the past decades, there are still diagnostic difficulty primarily due to the inability to always determine the pathogens. The interpretation of these potential pathogens remains challenging, because organism detection cannot always confirm the causation of infectious disease. For instance, multiplex PCRs for respiratory tract samples that include panels of viruses as well as bacterial and atypical pathogens are now being used to increase the etiological findings in LRTIs. The application of this technique has revealed high rates of coinfection, whereas the significance of which is still not clear. Further studies on the significance of these detected pathogens and their correlation with clinical findings are needed to help us differentiate colonization from infection. Certainly, with the increasing understanding of the respiratory microbiome, we may achieve greater insight into the etiology of LRTIs.

3   *Discussion*

A 22-year-old man had fever (38.5℃) for 3 days with cough and expectoration.

(1) Which kinds of diagnostic testing can be used for this case?

(2) If serum IgG of severe acute respiratory syndrome-related coronavirus-2 (SARS-CoV-2) is positive for this man, what do you think?

(3) If all the available tests are negative, should the infection be excluded?

References and resources

[1] JORGENSEN J H, PFALLER M A, CARROLL K C, et al. Manual of clinical microbiology [M]. 11th edition. Washington, D. C.: ASM press, 2015.

[2] KALIL A C, METERSKY M L, KLOMPAS M, et al. Management of adults with hospital-acquired and ventilator-associated pneumonia: 2016 clinical practice guidelines by the Infectious Diseases Society of America and the American Thoracic Society [J]. Clin Infect Dis, 2016, 63 (5): e61 – 111.

[3] YANG S, WU J, DING C, et al. Epidemiological features of and changes in incidence of infectious diseases in China in the first decade after the SARS outbreak: an observational trend study [J]. Lancet Infect Dis, 2017, 17 (7): 716 – 725.

[4] CAO B, HUANG Y, SHE D Y, et al. Diagnosis and treatment of community-acquired pneumonia in adults: 2016 clinical practice guidelines by the Chinese Thoracic Society, Chinese Medical Association [J]. Clin Respir J, 2018, 12 (4): 1320 – 1360.

(何　超)

CHAPTER 12

TUBERCULOSIS AND ITS DIAGNOSIS

1 *Words and phrases*

Acid-fast bacill'us 抗酸杆菌

Bacille Calmette-Guérin 卡介苗

Broth microdilution method 微量肉汤稀释法

Cavity 空洞

Extensively drug-resistant tuberculosis 泛耐药结核

Multidrug-resistant tuberculosis 多重耐药结核

Ethambutol 乙胺丁醇

Pyrazinamide 吡嗪酰胺

Rifampin 利福平

Fluorochrome stain 荧光染色

Interferon-γ release assay γ-干扰素释放试验

Immunochromatography 免疫色谱层析法

Isoniazid 异烟肼

Latent tuberculosis infection 潜伏性结核感染

Mycobacterium tuberculosis complex 结核分枝杆菌复合群

Mycobacterium leprae complex 麻风分枝杆菌复合群

Mycolic acid 分枝菌酸

Nontuberculous mycobacteria 非结核分枝杆菌

Oligonucleotide probe 寡核苷酸探针

PCR-reverse dot blot hybridization assay PCR 反向点杂交试验

Pleomorphic 多形性

Pulmonary tuberculosis 肺结核

Tuberculin skin test 结核菌素试验

Vaccine 疫苗

Ziehl-Neelsen stain 萋尼染色

2 Readings

2.1 Introduction

Within the genus *mycobacterium*, human pathogens consist of *Mycobacterium tuberculosis* complex (MTBC), *Mycobacterium leprae* complex and nontuberculous mycobacteria (NTM). Different species show various degrees of pathogenicity and virulence. After the HIV, the *Mycobacterium tuberculosis* complex is the second most important microorganisms that lead to a life-threatening infection in human beings.

2.1.1 *Mycobacterium tuberculosis* complex

The *Mycobacterium tuberculosis* complex, which include *M. tuberculosis*, *M. bovis*, *M. africanum*, *M. microti*, *M. canetti*, *M. caprae*, *M. pinnipedii*, and *M. orygis*, may invade any organ in the human body leading to chronic infection defined as tuberculosis (TB). The most commonly affecting organ is the lungs, followed by lymph nodes, pleura, bones, and joints. Tuberculosis affects men, women, and children in all age groups globally.

World Health Organization (WHO) reports 18 countries had more than 100 000 new cases with *M. tuberculosis* infection in 2016. The risk of developing TB is estimated to be between 16 – 27 times greater in people living with HIV than among those without HIV infection. In 2015, there were an estimated 10.4 million tuberculosis cases globally, including 1.2 million people living with HIV. Almost 60% of tuberculosis cases among people living with HIV were not diagnosed or treated, resulting in 390 000 tuberculosis related deaths among people living with HIV in 2015. WHO develops and promotes tools and guidelines to support countries in improving their TB/HIV collaborative action to achieve universal access to HIV and TB prevention, care and treatment services for all people in need. Additionally, drug-resistant tuberculosis is another challenge in the world. There were about 4.1% of newly infected patients and 19% previously treated patients resistant to rifampicin treatment in 2016 globally, among whom 490 000 (82%) cases were people with multidrug-resistant tuberculosis (resistant to rifampicin and isoniazid). Patients with multidrug-resistant tuberculosis are at high risk of treatment failure and new resistance to second-line drugs. Mortality from tuberculosis varies widely across the world, from less than 5% in some developed countries to more than 20% in most developing countries. India, Indonesia, China, Philippines, Pakistan, and most African countries, are tuberculosis high burden countries. In these countries, accurate diagnosis and appropriate chemotherapy for tuberculosis patients play a vital role in reducing human-to-human transmission and mortality rates.

M. tuberculosis is carried in droplet which is generated by patients with pulmonary tuberculosis coughing. Droplet inhalation is the most common human-to-human transmission mode. After inhalation, each individual may present different disease stages that depend on the host immune reaction. In most cases, *M. tuberculosis* could be eliminated via host immune system. However, in some cases, bacilli remain viable in the body. It can lead to primary progressive tuberculosis within 2 years of infection or latent tuberculosis infection (LTBI) with no clinical manifestations but tuberculin skin test (TST) or interferon-γ release assay (IGRA) positive.

2. 1. 2 *Mycobacterium leprae* complex

Mycobacterium leprae complex including *M. leprae* and *M. lepromatosis* causes the disease of leprosy which has clinical manifestations of the skin and peripheral nerves lesions. The number of newly diagnosed patients with leprosy was more than 210 000 worldwide in 2015, mostly reported from India, Brazil, Indonesia, and some African countries. Early diagnosis and appropriate treatment will help reduce the incidence of neurological deficits with mutilation.

The exact route of transmission of *Mycobacterium leprae* complex remains unclear. To date, droplet from the nasal mucosa is regarded as the most important transmission mode. Additionally, direct skin lesions contact with untreated, ulcerated, multibacillary lepromatous nodules is another possible transmission route.

2. 1. 3   Nontuberculous mycobacteria

Nontuberculous mycobacteria are ubiquitous in the natural environment and some species are conditional pathogens for human beings. Risk factors to infect NTM are as follows: pulmonary diseases like COPD, malignancy, immunosuppressive drugs, alcohol abuse, pneumoconiosis, and HIV infection. Several NTM species cause infection in humans, including *M. avium* complex, *M. kansasii*, *M. abscessus*, etc. There is no evidence of human-to-human transmission in patients with NTM infection.

2. 1. 4   Microbiological characteristics of Mycobacteria

Mycobacteria are non-motile, non-spore forming, pleomorphic, and Gram-positive bacilli. Most of the genus *mycobacterium* grow extremely slowly and its generation time is various from several hours to several days. The colony of mycobacteria on solid media is often wrinkled, pigmented, soft and buttery, smooth or rough, powdery to waxy, except that *Mycobacterium leprae* complex is unculturable in vitro.

The mycobacterial cell wall is rich in mycolic acid, which is usually resistant to decolorization by acidic ethanol in the Ziehl-Neelsen stain (Figure 12 - 1). The specific acid-fastness could help clinical microbiologists to differentiate mycobacteria from common bacteria under a microscope. Mycobacteria cells take up fuchsin or auramine O in phenol-water and then appear red (fuchsin stained) or exhibit yellow-green fluorescence (auramine O stained).

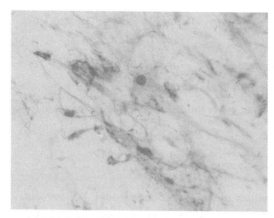

Figure 12 - 1   Ziehl-Neelsen stain of *Mycobacterium tuberculosis* (×1000).
(see Appendix Figure 19)

Rapid and reliable identification of *M. tuberculosis* complex is essential in a clinical microbiological laboratory. With the NTM species increased from 30 to more than 150, identification for NTM is another challenge for microbiologists. Phenotypic methods like the growth rate, optimal growth temperature, morphology, and pigmentation were pivotal for the successful identification of mycobacteria in the past few decades. However, these phenotypic methods are not accurate enough to discriminate a considerable amount of species of mycobacteria (Figure 12 - 2). Nowadays, nucleic acid detection is applied in clinical samples and could provide accurate results for identification.

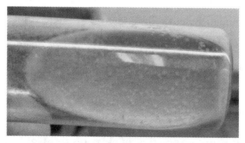

Figure 12 - 2   *Mycobacterium tuberculosis* grows on the Lowenstein-Jenden medium.
(see Appendix Figure 20)

2. 2   Diagnosis for tuberculosis

Diagnosis of tuberculosis can be made by clinical signs, chest X-ray finds, and laboratory examinations. Patients with active tuberculosis have clinical manifestations including fever (moderate, persistent 15 days or more), fatigue, weight loss, night sweats, loss of appetite, cough, hemoptysis, lymphadenopathy, and hepatosplenomegaly. In the cases with latent tuberculosis infection, patients have no clinical manifestation but may have exposure history and immunodiagnostic test (TST and IGRA) positive.

The radiological aspects in children under 10 years old show images with the primary complex of lungs. As the disease progresses, signs of imageology vary from person to person which include hilar lymphadenopathy, chronic or evolving pneumonia, and bilateral miliary pattern. The radiological aspects in most adults with primary progressive tuberculosis show apical posterior segment upper lobe infiltrates with or without a cavity, followed by lower lobe infiltrates, pulmonary nodules, pleural effusion, and hilar or paratracheal adenopathy. Patients with reactivation tuberculosis have typical apical cavities and secondary infiltrates in mid or lower lung fields. Other patterns include pleural tuberculosis, miliary, fibrotic apical scarring. Chest X-ray is essential for patients with suspected pulmonary tuberculosis.

Laboratory examination is the most important means for infection confirmation. Acid-fast bacilli discovered in clinical samples are strong evidence to confirm a patient with *M. tuberculosis* infection. Specific pathogen testing consists of direct microscopy, culture, nucleic acid detection. Sputum smear, a simple and rapid method for diagnosis, is widely applied to each patient with suspected active pulmonary tuberculosis in a medical institution, especially primary hospitals. And positive sputum (or other clinical samples) culture is a "gold standard" for the diagnosis of tuberculosis diseases. Moreover, cultures on the solid or broth media can be used for identification and antimicrobial susceptibility testing. Susceptibility testing of MTBC can be performed by the broth based method. When handling positive cultures with a high concentration of bacilli, skilled technologists and a safe laboratory environment with a good ventilation system are necessary for reducing cross contamination and aerosol transmission. However, biosafety level 3 facilities cannot be afforded in a most primary medical institute Therefore, sputum smear is still a significant method for the diagnosis of tuberculosis in most hospitals.

The nucleic acid test has been increasingly used in clinical specimens for MTBC detection. It takes only 2 hours to acquire results and could provide evidence for early diagnosis and treatment. With technological advances, the commercially available tests can be used for MTBC identification and susceptibility testing. For instance, the Xpert MTB/RIF test is available to detect MTBC nucleic acid and genome mutations associated with rifampin resistance via respiratory specimens.

The immunodiagnostic test includes tuberculin skin test and interferon-γ release assay. Tuberculin skin test had been widely used for screening tuberculosis infection in the past century. The purified protein derivative of tuberculin is injected intradermally into the volar aspect of the forearm. After 48 to 72 hours, an immune reaction is observed and induration is measured. It is noteworthy that people who previously received Bacille Calmette-Guérin (BCG) vaccine will show a positive reaction. In recent years, interferon-γ release assay (IGRA) is becoming a commonly immunodiagnostic test for tuberculosis. There are two methods to detect interferon-γ(IFN-γ) produced by activated T cells. In the first method, whole blood is added to a tube that is coated with the specific antigen of *M. tuberculosis* (ESAT-6 and CFP-10) and incubated for 24 hours. After that, plasma is separated and used for measuring the IFN-γ level.

The second method, an enzyme linked immunospot assay, is based on separating peripheral blood mononuclear cells (PBMCs) and incubating them with the specific antigens of *M. tuberculosis* (ESAT-6 and CFP-10) in a plate precoated with anti-IFN-γ antibodies for 20 hours. The positive results show visible spots and represent activated T cells. The method is commercially named T-SPOT assay.

The following part will take pulmonary tuberculosis as an example to illustrate the process of laboratory examination. Each means of laboratory examination for *M. tuberculosis* will be shown.

2.3 Case

A 34-year-old male patient was admitted with chief complaints of cough, fever, hemoptysis, and night sweats. Diagnosis of pulmonary tuberculosis was suspected by the physician-in-charge and then laboratory examination would need to be done to confirm the diagnosis.

2.3.1 Smear microscopy

Smear microscopy, as a rapid and simple method, is widely applied to diagnose tuberculosis in most medical institutes. According to the recommendation of ATS/CDC/IDSA, three sputum specimens should be collected 8 to 24 hours apart, which include at least an early morning specimen. Prepared sputum smears could be stained by the methods of auramine O-based fluorochrome stain or fuchsin-based Ziehl-Neelsen stain. On one hand, the fluorochrome stain has a higher sensitivity than the Ziehl-Neelsen stain because the fluorochrome-stained smears are easy to read. On the other hand, the fluorochrome stain has lower specificity than the Ziehl-Neelsen stain due to non-specific fluorescence existing. A combination of fluorochrome stain and Ziehl-Neelsen stain will contribute to improving the detection rate. Smear positive of auramine O stained specimens should be confirmed by the method of fuchsin-based Ziehl-Neelsen stain.

2.3.2 *M. tuberculosis* complex culture

For smear negative specimens, *M. tuberculosis* culture is more effective than smear microscopy because it can detect as few as 10^1 to 10^2 viable bacilli per milliliter. Media available for clinical specimens include solid and liquid ones. Lowenstein-Jenden medium, one the egg based solid media, is commonly used for mycobacteria culture which contains whole eggs or egg yolk, potato flour, salts, and glycerol. Apart from nutrients, an organic dyestuff of malachite green is added to the media for eliminating the growth of contaminating organisms. Middlebrook 7H9 broth is commonly used in the clinical microbiology laboratories. There are commercially automated, continuously monitoring systems developed for detecting the growth of mycobacteria, such as the Bactec MGIT 960 (Becton Dickinson). Both of them are broth media similar to Middlebrook 7H9 broth with additional various nutrients and antimicrobial agents. A fluorescence quenching-based oxygen sensor is utilized in the MGIT system to detect the signal of mycobacteria growth. Specimens are generally incubated for 6 to 8 weeks in liquid and on solid media before negative results are reported. Positive mycobacteria culture can be used for species identification and susceptibility testing. The information is pivotal to providing accurate diagnosis and treatment for patients.

2. 3. 3   *M. tuberculosis* complex identification

Once the culture is positive, a smear examination will be performed to confirm the isolates as acid-fast bacilli. And then it is essential to find out a rapid and accurate method for MTBC identification since the method of Ziehl-Neelsen stain cannot differentiate MTBC from other mycobacteria. In recent years, the immunochromatography based SD BIOLINE TB AgMPT64 RAPID test and protein mass fingerprinting based matrix assisted laser desorption ionization time-of-flight mass spectrometry (MALDI-TOF MS) have been developed and widely used for rapid MTBC identification.

MPT64, a specific antigen of TB bacteria, can be used to discriminate MTBC from NTM and BCG strains. Monoclonal mouse antibodies, against MPT64, are applied in the SD BIOLINE TB AgMPT64 RAPID test to detect MTBC. The test procedure is as follows. For cultures in liquid media, one hundred microliters of a sample are directly added to the sample well. For cultures on solid media, prepared suspension, 2 to 4 colonies suspended in extraction buffer, is added to the sample well like liquid media. After 15 minutes, the identification results are readable. If test and control lines are red, the test is positive; if only the control line is red, the test is negative; if only the test line is red, the test is invalid. This method provides rapid and reliable MTBC identification results after the culture is positive and could be widely used in primary medical institutes without any expensive equipment.

MALDI-TOF MS has been widely applied to varieties of microorganisms identification in recent years. Compared to the conventional methods, this technique is more rapid and accurate. Unlike most gram negative or positive bacteria, mycobacteria requires prior inactivation to reduce aerosol transmission and then cellular protein contents need to be released from the mycolic acid rich cell wall. Combined heat-killing, ethanol, sonication, and silica based bead beating with the routine formic acid/acetonitrile extraction is commonly recommended for mycobacteria inactivation and protein extracts in most situations. The protein extracts are spotted onto a polished steel target and mycobacteria identification is performed via mass spectrometry.

2. 3. 4   Immunodiagnostic testing

Tuberculin skin test (TST) is a common method to detect immune response after *M. tuberculosis* infection. Strong positive reaction with induration of 15mm or larger shows current infection with *M. tuberculosis* complex. A weak positive reaction means the subject is infected *with M. tuberculosis* complex or received BCG vaccination.

Interferon-γ release assay has been developed for the diagnosis of tuberculosis in recent years. Two specific antigens, early secreted antigenic target-6 (ESAT-6) and culture filtrate protein-10 (CFP-10), are encoded by a 9.5kb *M. tuberculosis* genomic segment which is absent from BCG and some environmental mycobacteria. Based on that, two methods previously described are used to detect IFN-γ level which can be used to diagnose latent *M. tuberculosis* infection.

2.3.5　Nucleic acid detection

Early detection of MTBC from clinical specimens is essential to provide a rapid result for accurate diagnosis and appropriate treatment. Direct nucleic acid detection technique for MTBC nucleic acid take only 2 hours to acquire results. The recommendation states that nucleic acid detection should be performed on at least one respiratory specimen from each patient suspected of pulmonary tuberculosis. The sensitivity and specificity of this technique are highest when smear-positive specimens are tested. Negative results of nucleic acid testing cannot rule out MTBC infection.

The Xpert MTB/RIF test is a newly developed commercial system to directly detect MTBC nucleic acid and mutations associated with rifampin resistance from clinical respiratory specimens. The WHO recommends that the Xpert MTB/RIF test should be performed in patients suspected of having multiple-drug-resistant or HIV associated tuberculosis. The method shows sensitivity of >70% in smear-negative specimens and a sensitivity of >90% in smear-positive specimens.

Resistance toward anti-TB drugs occurs mainly due to mutations in drug target genes. Previous studies show that more than 96% of the resistance inrifampin (RIF) is attributed to mutations in an 81 base pairs hot-spot pairs (codons 507 to 533) of the *rpoB* gene which encode the β-subunit of RNA polymerase. Among them, the most common mutations are observed in codons 531,526,516. High level isoniazid (INH) resistance is mainly associated with the mutations in the codon 315 of the *katG* gene which encodes the indispensable catalase-peroxidase enzyme for transforming INH into its active form. And low level INH resistance is mainly caused by the mutations in the −15 promoter region of the *inhA* gene which encodes enoyl-acyl carrier protein reductase. For ethambutol (EMB), the target is a key enzyme of arabinosyl transferases that is encoded by the *embCAB* operon and involved in the biosynthesis of arabinan, a critical component to form the cell wall. Mutations in the *embB* gene play a vital role in EMB resistance, especially in codon 306,406,497. Pyrazinamide (PZA) is activated by pyrazinamidase in the mycobacteria cell which is encoded by *pncA* gene. Unlike the first three drugs, resistance associated mutations in *pncA* are dispersed along the whole gene segment without any hot-spot regions. With the process of science and technology, a number of genotypic assays have been developed for drug susceptibility testing, including DNA sequencing, polymerase chain reaction single stranded conformational polymorphism, and PCR-reverse dot blot hybridization assay. Among these technologies, PCR reverse dot blot hybridization assay has been commercially applied to detect *M. tuberculosis* resistance in clinical respiratory specimens. In the method, oligonucleotide probes based on wild and mutant genotype sequences (*rpoB* for RIF, *katG*, and *inhA* for INH, *embB* for EMB, *pncA* for PZA) are designed to detect common resistance associated mutations to indicate drug resistance. Many special oligonucleotide probes are coated in the negatively charged nylon membrane. According to the complementary nature of the base pairs, PCR products from clinical specimens will bind to some special oligonucleotide probes and then the mutant genotype of the *M. tuberculosis* can be acquired after several hours. Rapid susceptibility testing results for the four first line drugs will contribute to optimizing the appropriate therapies and improving outcome for patients with multidrug-resistant tuberculosis. In addition, metagenomic next-generation sequencing (mNGS) are also widely used in the diagnosis of tuberculosis.

All in all, nucleic acid detection provides rapid and accurate identification and susceptibility testing results for the diagnosis of tuberculosis, but it cannot replace the conventional methods like mycobacteria culture and phenotypic drug susceptibility testing.

2.3.6   Phenotypic drug susceptibility testing

The emergence of multidrug-resistant TB (MDR-TB) and extensively drug-resistant TB (XDR-TB) poses a risk to TB control and treatment worldwide. Treatment of MDR/XDR TB is complicated and requires a long duration with a combination of at least four drugs. Phenotypic drug susceptibility testing is essential to provide accurate information for MDR/XDR therapy. The following antibiotics are tested during the same time: rifampin, rifabutin, isoniazid, ethambutol, pyrazinamide, capreomycin, ofloxacin, levofloxacin, moxifloxacin, kanamycin, amikacin, para-aminosalicylic acid, streptomycin. The procedure of drug susceptibility testing for MTBC is similar to the broth microdilution method of common bacteria except that the former will take a few weeks rather than 18 to 20 hours. Prepared suspension is added to wells that are precoated with antibiotics. After 6 days, daily observation will need to be performed by experienced technologists. Phenotypic drug susceptibility testing results can be acquired after 2 to 3 weeks.

2.3.7   Routine laboratory testing

Routing laboratory testing including complete blood count, HIV testing, transaminase testing, creatinine level, and glomerular filtration rate is not diagnostic, but it provides clues to diagnose disease and serves as a baseline against which to monitor response to treatment and drug toxicities. Patients with *M. tuberculosis* infection may present anemia of chronic disease and high level transaminase after anti-TB drugs treatment. Routine laboratory testing will help formulate appropriate therapies for patients with tuberculosis.

In conclusion, laboratory examination of *M. tuberculosis* is indispensable to provide bacterial evidence for tuberculosis diagnosis. According to " the WHO Treatment of Tuberculosis Guideline (the fourth edition)", a patient with one positive acid-fastness bacilli is regarded as a definite case in countries with a functional external quality assurance system. For smear-negative TB, it is pivotal to combine laboratory examination with clinical manifestation, chest X-ray finding, and immunodiagnostic testing to diagnose and evaluate the degree of illness.

3 *Discussion*

(1) A 22-year-old male patient complains that he has coughed with sputum and blood for 4 months, what laboratory examination should be done for him?

(2) A young male patient who had been diagnosed with pulmonary tuberculosis has received anti-TB drugs for three months, but now sputum smear from the patient is still positive for acid-fast bacilli. Next, what examination should be done for him?

(3) A 39-year-old female patient complains about shortness of breath and cough with sputum. She has received renal transplantation for three years. And then, what examination should be done for her?

Reference and resources

[1] FLOYD K, GLAZIOU P, ZUMLA A, et al. The global tuberculosis epidemic and progress in care, prevention, and research: an overview in year 3 of the end TB era [J]. The Lancet Respiratory Medicine, 2018, 6 (4): 299 – 314.

[2] BLUMBERG H M, BURMAN W J, CHAISSON R E, et al. American Thoracic Society/Centers for Disease Control and Prevention/Infectious Diseases Society of America: treatment of tuberculosis [J]. American journal of respiratory and critical care medicine, 2003, 167 (4): 603 – 662.

[3] JORGENSEN J H, PFALLER M A, CARROLL K C, et al. Manual of clinical microbiology (2 Volume set) [M]. 11th ed. Washington DC: ASM press, 2015.

[4] BANSAL R, SHARMA D, SINGH R. Tuberculosis and its treatment: an overview [J]. Mini reviews in medicinal chemistry, 2018, 18 (1): 58 – 71.

[5] FISCHER M. Leprosy-an overview of clinical features, diagnosis, and treatment [J]. Journal of the German Society of Dermatology, 2017, 15 (8): 801 – 827.

[6] BARKSDALE L, KIM K S. Mycobacterium [J]. Bacteriological reviews, 1977, 41 (1): 217 – 372.

[7] Carvalho A C C, Cardoso C A A, Martire TM, et al. Epidemiological aspects, clinical manifestations, and prevention of pediatric tuberculosis from the perspective of the End

TB Strategy [J]. Jornal brasileiro de pneumologia, 2018, 44 (2): 134 – 144.

[8] SIA I G, WIELAND M L. Current concepts in the management of tuberculosis [J].
Mayo Clinic proceedings, 2011, 86 (4): 348 – 361.

[9] SOYSAL A, BAKIR M. T-SPOT. TB assay usage in adults and children [J]. Expert
review of molecular diagnostics, 2011, 11 (6): 643 – 660.

[10] LEWINSOHN D M, LEONARD M K, LOBUE P A, et al. Official American Thoracic
Society/Infectious Diseases Society of America/Centers for Disease Control and
Prevention clinical practice guidelines: diagnosis of tuberculosis in adults and children
[J]. Clinical infectious diseases, 2017, 64 (2): 111 – 115.

[11] SHENOY V P, MUKHOPADHYAY C. Rapid immunochromatographic test for the
identification and discrimination of mycobacterium tuberculosis complex isolates from
non-tuberculous mycobacteria [J]. Journal of clinical and diagnostic research, 2014,
8 (4): DC13 – 15.

[12] CEYSSENS P J, SOETAERT K, TIMKE M, et al. Matrix-assisted laser desorption
ionization-time of flight mass spectrometry for combined species identification and drug
sensitivity testing in mycobacteria [J]. Journal of clinical microbiology, 2017, 55
(2): 624 – 634.

[13] GUO Q, YU Y, ZHU Y L, et al. Rapid detection of rifampin-resistant clinical isolates
of Mycobacterium tuberculosis by reverse dot blot hybridization [J]. Biomedical and
environmental sciences, 2015, 28 (1): 25 – 35.

[14] WU X, ZHANG J, CHAO L, et al. Identification of rifampin-resistant genotypes in
Mycobacterium tuberculosis by PCR-reverse dot blot hybridization [J]. Molecular
biotechnology, 2009, 41 (1): 1 – 7.

[15] UNISSA A N, SUBBIAN S, HANNA L E, et al. Overview on mechanisms of isoniazid
action and resistance in Mycobacterium tuberculosis [J]. Journal of molecular
epidemiology and evolutionary genetics in infectious diseases, 2016, 45: 474 – 492.

[16] NACHAPPA S A, NEELAMBIKE S M, AMRUTHAVALLI C, et al. Detection of first-
line drug resistance mutations and drug-protein interaction dynamics from tuberculosis
patients in South India [J]. Microbial drug resistance, 2018, 24 (4): 377 – 385.

[17] SUN Q, XIAO T Y, LIU H C, et al. Mutations within embCAB are associated with
variable level of ethambutol resistance in mycobacterium tuberculosis isolates from China
[J]. Antimicrob Agents Chemother, 2018, 62 (1): e01279 – 17.

[18] TAM K K, LEUNG K S, SIU G K, et al. Direct detection of pyrazinamide resistance
of Mycobacterium tuberculosis using pncA PCR sequencing [J]. Journal of clinical
microbiology, 2019, 57 (8): e00145 – 19.

[19] SURESH N, SINGH U B, ARORA J, et al. Rapid detection of rifampicin-resistant
Mycobacterium tuberculosis by in-house, reverse line blot assay [J]. Diagnostic

microbiology and infectious disease, 2006, 56 (2): 133 – 140.

[20] HEYCKENDORF J, ANDRES S, KOSER C U, et al. What is resistance? impact of phenotypic versus molecular drug resistance testing on therapy for multi-and extensively drug-resistant tuberculosis [J]. Antimicrob Agents Chemother, 2018, 62 (2): e01550 – 17.

（谢　轶）